The Athletic Trainer's Guide to Strength and Endurance Training

The Athletic Trainer's Guide to Strength and Endurance Training

Denise Wiksten, PhD, ATC
San Diego State University
San Diego, California

Carolyn Peters, MA, ATC, CSCS
San Diego State University
San Diego, California

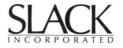

SLACK
INCORPORATED

6900 Grove Road • Thorofare, NJ 08086

Publisher: John H. Bond
Editorial Director: Amy E. Drummond
Editorial Assistant: William J. Green

The work SLACK Incorporated publishes is peer reviewed. Prior to publication, recognized leaders in the field, educators, and clinicians provide important feedback on the concepts and content that we publish. We welcome feedback on this work.

Wiksten, Denise L.
  The athletic trainer's guide to strength and endurance training / Denise Wiksten,
Carolyn Peters.
     p. cm.
  Includes bibliographical references (p.) and index.
  ISBN 1-55642-431-0 (alk. paper)
  1. Sports--Physiological aspects. 2. Muscle strength. 3. Physical fitness. 4. Physical education and training. I. Peters, Carolyn, II. Title.

RC1235 . W56 2000
613.7'11--dc21

                                                        00-041326

Printed in the United States of America.
Published by: SLACK Incorporated
                       6900 Grove Road
                       Thorofare, NJ 08086 USA
                       Telephone: 856-848-1000
                       Fax: 856-853-5991
                       www.slackbooks.com

Last digit is print number: 10 9 8 7 6 5 4 3 2 1

DEDICATION

To Eric, Annamarie, and EJ for your support, unconditional love, and inspiration.
Denise Wiksten

To the memory of Mom and Dad. To Janet and Susan, my best friends who happen to be my sisters; and David, my friend and mentor, for all of their strength and guidance.
Carolyn Peters

CONTENTS

Section 5: Injury Prevention and Management Techniques

Section 6: Sport-Specific Strength Training Programs

ACKNOWLEDGMENTS

The completion of this book could not have been accomplished without the assistance of David Ohton, Bob Moore, Janis Badolato, Eileen Bermundo, Tom Farrington, Larry Verity, Jeanne Nichols, and Ed Franz. We would like to express our sincere thanks to these individuals for their support and guidance. In addition, we would like to thank Marje Albohm and SLACK, Inc. for their insight into the potential of this textbook and its inclusion in the *Athletic Training Library* series.

ABOUT THE AUTHORS

Denise Wiksten is an Associate Professor in the Department of Exercise and Nutritional Sciences at San Diego State University. She is also the Program Director of the CAAHEP accredited Athletic Training Program at San Diego State University. She received her PhD in Sports Medicine from the University of Virginia in 1994. Work from her dissertation examined the relationship between muscle strength and balance as a function of age. The results of this research can be found in the international journal, *Isokinetic Science and Exercise.* Subsequently, her research efforts have centered on balance and muscle performance testing in a variety of age groups and populations. She has also focused her research interests in the area of multimedia education and the effects of classroom integration. She is the co-author of the textbook, *Special Tests for Orthopedic Examination* and has authored a multimedia two-disc series titled, *Upper and Lower Extremity Injury Evaluation: An Interactive Approach.*

Carolyn Peters began her career in strength and conditioning as a Division 1 shot putter and basketball player. After a successful career at San Diego State University, she became a Certified Athletic Trainer and Certified Strength and Conditioning Specialist. Working as an assistant strength and conditioning coach at SDSU for 3 years gave her the opportunity to work closely with, and instruct, both men's and women's varsity and club teams. An abstract of her Master's thesis, *A Comparison of Two Basketball Specific Stretching Programs on Vertical Jumping Ability and Incidence of Injury* was published in *The Basketball Bulletin.* She was selected to participate on an expert panel for the evaluation of United States Marine Corp recruit training in San Diego, where the panel created recommendations for modifying the USMC recruit-training program to reduce military training related injuries. Recently Carolyn instructed approximately 400 firefighters and paramedics on *Strength Training and Core Stabilization for Job Performance and Injury Reduction.* Currently she is working as a Certified Athletic Trainer at San Diego State University.

CONTRIBUTING AUTHOR

Mark Kern is a Registered Dietitian and an assistant professor in the Department of Exercise and Nutritional Sciences at San Diego State University in San Diego, CA. He received his PhD in Foods and Nutrition from Purdue University. Mark has taught many nutrition courses and regularly teaches a *Nutrition for Athletes* class. He also directs nutrition consulting with the varsity athletes at San Diego State along with the Head Athletic Trainer. His research interests include sports nutrition research and the effects of diet and exercise on risk for chronic diseases such as heart disease and osteoporosis.

PREFACE

As Certified Athletic Trainers, it is crucial that we have and continue to employ people with a multifaceted educational background. Areas often neglected are those of administration, nutrition, needs of our special populations, and strength and endurance training. The registered dietitian, the certified strength and conditioning specialist, and those who are certified by other allied health professional organizations are those who should be employed to fill the need in these areas. Unfortunately, not all levels of athletic participation are fortunate enough to have these proficient individuals easily accessible to the participant. Fortunately, the curricula of today's athletic trainer includes many courses on these specialties. Certified Athletic Trainers who work with young high school athletes often find themselves as the acting nutritionist or strength training professional. How often has a coach inquired about a stretching or circuit program the day before practice is to begin? Will you know the appropriate spotting procedures or weight lifting techniques for your more progressed athletes? Are you able to respond when a team inquires about a healthy eating plan? These are all ways we as Certified Athletic Trainers can contribute to the prevention of sports injuries. Even at the collegiate level, a working knowledge of these domains is very advantageous as we accelerate the athlete through his/her rehabilitation program. It is especially important to incorporate total body wellness, strength, and endurance training as the athlete progresses through the return to activity phase during rehabilitation. One of the most discouraging aspects of our profession is to rehabilitate athletes only to have them fail due to inadequate energy levels, poor cardiovascular conditioning, or lack of maintained strength.

This book will offer the appropriate tools for you to understand and implement the domains of strength training, speed training, plyometrics, endurance training, nutritional aids for sport performance, injury prevention, and needs for special populations. Rather than read from cover to cover, locate your desired topic in the table of contents and review that specific section. The text is meant for review. For example, prior to implementing a lower extremity plyometric program, you may wish to review Chapter Six which deals with the principles of plyometrics. The supplemental and sport-specific programs presented in Section 6 are designed for quick use. The sports are in alphabetical order and the program phases are in proper sequence.

Remember, while we cannot be all things to all people all the time, we can strive to expand our knowledge, rely on useful references, and refer to appropriate specialists when necessary.

FOREWORD

Over the past 10 years, athletes and the competitive sports in which they play have reached new levels of sophistication. During that same time period, the demands on the athletic trainer to provide a higher level of quality sports health care have also increased. The increases in sophistication of physical conditioning have demanded greater attention in the area of injury prevention. One particular facet of sport injury prevention involves knowledge of strength and endurance conditioning.

The timing of Wiksten and Peters' book titled *The Athletic Trainers Guide to Strength and Endurance Training* is very appropriate. This book is a beneficial and realistic guide for the athletic trainer, whether involved in the development of a strength and conditioning program, consultation with the strength and conditioning staff, or developing and supervising clinical rehabilitation protocols. This book is written by athletic trainers for athletic trainers. It provides the reader with the necessary theoretical and physiological foundation, while at the same time enabling the clinician the opportunity to "put into practice" very useful and easy to understand strength and conditioning techniques. Wiksten and Peters should be commended for having the foresight to see that this is one area in which an athletic trainer needs useful and practical knowledge to carry out a well-rounded sports health care delivery program.

Readers should find the section on "Nutritional Aids for Sports Performance," containing important information on optimal diets for sport performance and supplements for strength and endurance, especially appealing. They present information that is not only relevant, but very contemporary too. Another section titled "Sport-Specific Strength Training Programs" contains very detailed strength and conditioning programs for a variety of sporting activities. These programs should help the athletic trainer/clinician develop a foundation from which to initiate athletic conditioning programs.

Wiksten and Peters have assembled a very user-friendly textbook that should become part of every athletic trainer's personal library. This book is equally thought provoking and informative and will provide clinicians with the necessary background information to strengthen their skills in the area of strength and conditioning.

Tom Kaminski, PhD, ATC/L

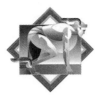

Section 1

Introduction

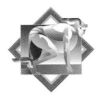 Chapter One

Historical Perspectives of Related Professional Organizations

The following information on the various professional organizations and certifying committees has been compiled based upon information gained directly from the internet and brochures published by the respective organization. Contact information for each organization is also provided.

NATIONAL STRENGTH AND CONDITIONING ASSOCIATION (NSCA)

1955 N. Union Boulevard
Colorado Springs, CO 80909
Phone: (719) 632-6722
Fax: (719) 632-6367
Email: nsca@usa.net
Website: http://www.nsca-lift.org/

NSCA Mission Statement

"The National Strength and Conditioning Association, as a non-profit, worldwide authority on strength and conditioning for improved physical and athletic performance, creates and disseminates related knowledge and enhances the careers of its members."

Membership

The NSCA provides its members with a wide variety of resources and opportunities designed to enhance their education and careers. Members have access to the latest research findings, breakthrough techniques, and the most up-to-date conditioning practices and injury prevention methods.

Certifications

Credentialing for the strength and conditioning specialist was initiated in 1985 as a way to identify and recognize those professionals who possess the knowledge to design and implement safe and effective strength training and conditioning programs. The NSCA Certification Commission now offers two certification programs, the Certified Strength and Conditioning Specialist (CSCS) and the NSCA-Certified Personal Trainer (NSCA-CPT). CSCS professionals primarily educate and train athletes in proper strength and conditioning practices. They work in a variety of settings including educational institutions, sports medicine clinics, health and fitness clubs, and corporate wellness centers.

NSCA-CPTs train clients in a one-on-one situation in the client's home, health and fitness clubs, and YMCAs. Personal trainers often specialize their expertise to accommodate clients with difficulties such as orthopedic, cardiovascular, or weight problems, as well as other chronic conditions. They also work with the physically impaired and the elderly.

In order to be eligible for certification, one must hold a bachelor's degree, or be enrolled as a college senior at an accredited college or university. One must also be CPR certified and must pass the certification examination.

For more information on certification, you may contact the NSCA Certification Commission at:

NSCA Certification Commission
1640 "L" Street, Suite G
Lincoln, NE 68508
Phone: (402) 476-6669
Toll free: (888) 746-2378
Fax: (402) 476-7141
Website: http://www.nsca-lift.org/

AMERICAN COLLEGE OF SPORTS MEDICINE (ACSM)

P.O. Box 1440
Indianapolis, IN 46206
Phone: (317) 637-9200
Fax: (317) 634-7817
Website: http://www.acsm.org/

ACSM Mission Statement

"The American College of Sports Medicine promotes and integrates scientific research, education, and practical applications of sports medicine and exercise science to maintain and enhance physical performance, fitness, health, and quality of life."

Position Statement

The ACSM has an official position statement titled, "The Recommended Quantity and Quality of Exercise for Developing and Maintaining Cardiorespiratory and Muscular Fitness in Healthy Adults." It can be found in the official journal for the ACSM, *Medicine and Science in Sports and Exercise*, Volume 22, pages 265-274, 1990.

Membership

There are a variety of membership categories with the ACSM. The following list identifies each of the member types.

PROFESSIONAL MEMBER:

This category is open to anyone who has earned a bachelor's, master's, or doctoral degree at an accredited institution in a field related to health, physical education, or exercise science; or anyone who has earned at least a bachelor's degree in another area but is working in a field related to sports medicine or exercise science.

PROFESSIONAL MEMBER-IN-TRAINING:

Professional-in-training membership is limited only to physicians in residency or postdoctoral fellows.

GRADUATE STUDENT MEMBER:

This category is open to any student who has earned a bachelor's degree in a field related to exercise science or sports medicine and is carrying at least one-half of a full academic load, as defined by the attending institution, during at least one semester of a regular academic year.

UNDERGRADUATE STUDENT MEMBER:

This category is open to any full-time undergraduate student studying in a field related to exercise science or sports medicine.

ASSOCIATE MEMBER:

Associate membership is open to anyone with an interest in the general area of sports medicine or exercise science but who does not possess at least a bachelor's degree and does not qualify for any other category of membership (excluding the ACSM Alliance of Health & Fitness Professionals).

ACSM's ALLIANCE OF HEALTH & FITNESS PROFESSIONALS:

Alliance membership is open to anyone with an interest in health and fitness issues.

Certifications

ACSM offers different levels of certification within two specific tracks.

HEALTH & FITNESS TRACK CERTIFICATIONS INCLUDE:

- ACSM Exercise Leader

- ACSM Health/Fitness Instructor
- ACSM Health/Fitness Director

These certifications are available if you are involved with fitness in a setting where the exercise participants are apparently healthy and are exercising for health maintenance.

CLINICAL TRACK CERTIFICATIONS INCLUDE:

- ACSM Exercise Specialist
- ACSM Exercise Test Technologist
- ACSM Program Director

These certifications are designed for those individuals who work in clinical settings where the participants are engaged in cardiac or pulmonary rehabilitation or have a chronic disease such as diabetes.

In addition, ASCM offers any certified member the opportunity to earn a certificate of enhanced qualification (CEQ). These include:

- ACSM Advanced Personal Trainer CEQ
- ACSM Exercise and the Older Adult CEQ
- ACSM Nutrition and Exercise: From Health to Physical Performance CEQ

NATIONAL ATHLETIC TRAINERS' ASSOCIATION (NATA)

2952 Stemmons Freeway
Dallas, TX 75247-6196
Phone: (214) 637-6282
Toll free: (800) TRY-NATA
Fax: (214) 637-2206
Website: http://www.nata.org

NATA Mission Statement

"The mission of the National Athletic Trainers' Association is to enhance the quality of health care for athletes and those engaged in physical activity, and to advance the profession of athletic training through education and research in the prevention, evaluation, management and rehabilitation of injuries."

Position Statements

The NATA has issued official statements on the following topics:

- Physically Active Definition
- Blood Borne Pathogens Guidelines
- Secondary School Athletic Trainers
- Recommendations for the Appropriate Care of the Spine-Injured Athlete
- Guidelines for the Pre-hospital Management of Suspected Spinal Injury

The actual statements appear on the NATA website or can be requested in writing from the NATA national office.

Membership

The membership year is January 1 through December 31. The annual membership fee consists of a national fee and a district fee (with the exception of supplier members, who do not have district affiliation). Individuals may apply for NATA membership in one of the following categories:

CERTIFIED MEMBER:

This membership category is open only to individuals possessing current National Athletic Trainers' Board of Certification (NATABOC) certification. Certified membership has four subcategories:

- Regular
- Graduate student
- International
- Retired

ASSOCIATE MEMBER:

This membership category is open to individuals who are working professionally in athletics, education, research, medicine, or an allied health or other profession related to athletic training.

STUDENT MEMBER:

- This membership category is open only to individuals meeting one of the criteria below:
- Noncertified individuals enrolled as full-time graduate students in an accredited college or university.
- Individuals currently making progress toward the fulfillment of the requirements for NATABOC certification by participating in an internship or approved curriculum program under the supervision of an NATABOC certified athletic trainer.

INTERNATIONAL MEMBER:

This membership category is open only to non-certified individuals who do not have a permanent address in the United States or Canada. Members of this category are not eligible for district affiliation and may not vote or hold office in the NATA. Individuals who are stationed temporarily overseas with the military are not eligible for membership in this category.

SUPPLIER MEMBER:

This membership category is open only to corporations, which are suppliers and/or manufacturers of athletic training materials, supplies, equipment, or services. Each supplier member will be entitled to designate one individual as the corporation's representative to the NATA. Members of this category are not eligible for district affiliation and may not vote or hold office within the NATA. Supplier members will be entitled to member discount rates on a variety of products and services, including reduced advertising rates on NATA's publications and reduced exhibit booth rental fees at the annual meeting.

Certification

NATABOC was incorporated in 1989 to provide a certification program for entry-level athletic trainers and recertification standards for Certified Athletic Trainers. The purpose of this entry-level certification program is to establish standards for entry into the profession of athletic training. Additionally, the NATABOC has established the continuing education requirements that Certified Athletic Trainers must satisfy in order to maintain status as a NATABOC certified athletic trainer.

Currently there are two routes to certification for the athletic trainer:
- Internship route
- Accredited program route

As of January 1, 2004, the only route to certification will be through an accredited athletic training education program. The requirements for candidacy for the NATABOC Certification Examination are available by contacting the NATABOC at:

1512 S. 60th Street
Omaha, NE 68106
Phone: 877-BOC-EXAM
Fax: 402-561-0598
E-mail: staff@nataboc.org
Web site: http://www.nataboc.org

AMERICAN COUNCIL ON EXERCISE (ACE)

5820 Oberlin Drive, Suite 102
San Diego, CA 92121-3787
Phone: (619) 535-8227
Fax: (619) 535-1778
Web site: http://acefitness.org

ACE Mission Statement

> *"The American Council on Exercise (ACE) is a nonprofit organization committed to promoting active, healthy lifestyles and their positive effects on the mind, body and spirit. ACE pledges to enable all segments of society to enjoy the benefits of physical activity and protect the public against unsafe and ineffective fitness products and trends. ACE accomplishes this mission by setting certification and education standards for fitness instructors and through ongoing public education about the importance of exercise."*

Membership

Becoming ACE certified entitles the member to many benefits. ACE offers a complete referral service and consultant bureau for its members. Members also have the opportunity to attend continuing education courses that enable them to continue scientific inquiry into the health and fitness arena.

Certification

ACE offers the following certifications:

PERSONAL TRAINER:

Certified Personal Trainers work with individuals who need expertise on exercise physiology, kinesiology, nutrition, fitness assessment, exercise programming, etc.

CLINICAL EXERCISE SPECIALIST:

Clinical Exercise Specialists help bridge the gap between the healthcare industry and the health club. Specifically, they are able to help people who have received treatment or rehabilitation for a health challenge and have been cleared for exercise by their physicians.

GROUP FITNESS INSTRUCTOR:

Group Fitness Instructors are certified to lead groups in aerobic-style movements; and apply knowledge of anatomy, kinesiology, exercise physiology, instructional techniques, and injury prevention.

LIFESTYLE & WEIGHT MANAGEMENT CONSULTANT:

Lifestyle & Weight Management Consultants, combine the sciences of exercise and nutrition with lifestyle changes to make a difference in the daily lives of the average population.

Before taking any ACE certification examination:
1. You must be at least 18 years of age.
2. You must have current adult CPR (cardiopulmonary resuscitation) certification. Your CPR certification must be current at the time of the exam. CPR certifications are accepted from the following organizations:
    - American Heart Association (or international equivalent)
    - American Red Cross (or international equivalent)
    - Medic First Aid (PADI)
    - Emergency Medical Technician (EMT)

Once certified, ACE offers the opportunity for Specialty Recognition Certificates in the following areas.
- Aquatic exercise
- Flexibility training
- Pre/Postnatal fitness
- Boxing aerobics
- Indoor cycling
- Step/bench exercise

- Exercise-ball training
- Mind/body integration
- Strength training
- Fitness business
- Nutrition
- Walking fitness
- Fitness management
- Older adult fitness
- Youth fitness

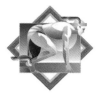

Chapter Two

Safety and Legal Issues

Before you embark on your journey of becoming a resourceful professional, it is encouraged and highly recommended that you investigate the legalities surrounding the implementation of the suggestions in this book. The advice of professional legal counsel is the first step to ensuring a safe and effective atmosphere for everyone involved. During your legal consultation, focus should be on liability insurance, waivers, and assumption of risk documents. The magnitude of the consequences of neglect in these areas can be very costly and disrupting for you and your employer. Waivers, assumption of risk documents, and the like, should be signed prior to the facility orientation and kept on file. Your legal counsel should determine the length of keeping said documents.

In California, (Sanchez vs. Bally's Total Fitness Corp., Case Number B116567, [Court of Appeals, Second Appellate District, 1998]) a popular health club was protected from a costly lawsuit by having a signed release on file. The member was injured during a break in her aerobics class and was claiming negligence against the club for not instructing her on proper equipment break down and storage. She claimed the signed release did not contain the word "negligence," therefore it was nonspecific and void. The court claimed that the intent of the document was to release the club of responsibility due to injuries sustained during use of the equipment and its facility. The importance of keeping signed waivers and release forms is apparent in this case. A small investment of time and money may turn out to be very beneficial in the long run.

Once you have secured the applicable legal documents for your state, extensive attention should be given to the emergency management plan. The verdict of a recent lawsuit supports this suggestion. The case, Spiegler vs. State of Arizona (Maricopa County Supreme Court, Arizona, Case No. CV92-13608, 1996) involved a 21-year-old female student at the University of Arizona. She had been diagnosed with hypertrophic cardiomyopathy and was exercising under the recommendation of a physician. During a routine workout, she suffered a cardiac arrest. The staff was instructed, through their policies and procedures, to administer CPR as necessary. The supervising student employee failed to do so but did call 911. Due to this insubordination, the impaired young woman suffered permanent brain damage. The jury found in favor of the plaintiff, not for having suffered the cardiac arrest in the facility, but for not being given the adequate standard of care previously determined by the facility's policies and procedures. So, not only is it important to have a detailed emergency care plan, but it is imperative that supervisors and employees be educated in the plan and follow it accordingly.

Spotting a weightlifter may be another area taken for granted, yet this must not be overlooked in the legal arena. According to the National Strength and Conditioning Association, it is the duty of the spotter to inspect the area around the lifter. It must be free of debris and provide enough space between the lifters and equipment. In a recent case from the Superior Court of New Jersey (Parks vs. Gilligan, Law Division, Ocean County, docket #OCN-L-1945-96), a spotter and the facility were found liable for the plaintiff's damaged finger. The plaintiff lowered his dumbbells after completing the lift and crushed a finger between a dumbbell and a weight on the floor. Apparently, the spotter and the staff were not aware of the weight being in the proximity of the lifter but were found partially responsible for negligence regardless.

In a case from Ohio (Sicard vs. University of Dayton, reported at 104 Ohio Appellate 3d 27, 1995), the plaintiff claimed his spotters failed to assist with a heavy bench press repetition that subsequently resulted in a major injury. Although the court concluded that weightlifting has its risks of potential injury merely due to the nature of the sport, it did not concur that participants should be subject to failing weights or equipment. Therefore, the plaintiff was granted restitution.

Spotting is part of a standard of care, and spotters should take this duty seriously and ensure that the service is adequately provided. The facility and its supervisors should take the responsibility of educating and providing acceptable spotting coverage. Suggestions on proper spotting techniques will be discussed in Section 5, Injury Prevention and Management Techniques.

The following are some basic suggestions for any facility and staff.

FACILITY

- Limit occupant capacity to avoid overcrowding.
- Space equipment adequately (2 to 3 ft. between each apparatus).
- Confirm adequate height space for platform area (12 to 15 ft.).
- Section off specific areas, eg, platforms, dumbbells, barbells, machines etc.
- Keep walkways and entrances free from debris.
- Post facility hours of operation.
- Post emergency care plan.
- Post warning signs of overexertion.
- Post facility rules and regulations.
- Keep facility clean, well lighted, and at a comfortable temperature.
- Adequate restroom facilities should be available.
- Keep water cooler (suggest using cone cups) separate and clear from equipment.

STAFF

- Make all employees aware of plans, policies, and procedures.
- Employ professionals certified by an accredited association.
- Certify all employees in CPR and First Aid.
- Complete health questionnaire, eg, Personal Activity Readiness Questionnaire (PAR-Q).
- Educate in correct lifting and spotting techniques.
- Practice the emergency plan every quarter.
- Routinely inspect facility and equipment.
- Document and report any defects or possible dangers.
- Keep equipment clean and schedule regular maintenance checks.
- Maintain an appropriate number of supervisors.
- Maintain signed legal documents.

PARTICIPANTS

- Schedule an orientation for equipment usage and lifting techniques.
- Dress in appropriate attire and footwear.
- Use of a spotter is recommended.
- Restack and replace all weights.
- Horseplay or profanity will not be tolerated.
- The use of personal portable radios is prohibited.
- Keep personal items out of facility.
- Food, gum, drinks, tobacco, toothpicks etc, are prohibited.
- Follow the guidance and instruction of supervisors.

In conclusion, the authors wish to stress the importance of consulting a legal professional, implementing and following through with an emergency management plan, and detailing policies and procedures for the facility, staff, and its participants.

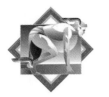

Section 2

Strength Training

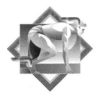 Chapter Three

Principles of Human Muscle Performance

Human muscle performance is the ability of a muscle to produce force. This is dependent upon specific anatomical and physiological characteristics of the muscle that are beyond the scope of this book. This chapter focuses specifically on the types of muscle performance and biomechanical factors that affect strength training. When a muscle contracts, physiological adaptations occur that result in force development within the muscle. This contraction may result in a shortening of the muscle, lengthening of the muscle, or no change in length of the muscle, depending on the type of external force applied. The following principles describe the different mechanisms of human muscle performance and will provide a basis for the following chapters that focus on specific strength training techniques.

ISOMETRIC MUSCLE PERFORMANCE

During an isometric contraction, the muscle contracts and produces a static force with no change in joint angle or muscle length. It is a method of assessing maximum static force as well as exercising the muscle when joint range of motion is contraindicated. Other advantages of this type of exercise and muscle performance assessment technique are that it requires minimal or no equipment to perform, and can be performed anywhere. For example, contracting the deltoid muscle by attempting to abduct the arm while standing against a wall or in a doorway allows for increased muscle tension in the deltoid muscle at that specified length and position. Similarly, the biceps muscle can be exercised isometrically by positioning the hand under a desk or countertop and lifting upward against the resistance of the static desk or countertop. The use of cable tensiometry and dynamometers allows for measurement of isometric muscle performance. The disadvantages of this type of exercise is that the muscle is trained only at the specific joint angle at which it is being exercised or assessed, it is difficult to assess increases in strength, and there is less of objective feedback as compared to isotonic and isokinetic muscle performance.

Isotonic Muscle Performance

During an isotonic muscle contraction, force from a muscle action overcomes some form of fixed external resistance while the joint moves throughout the range of motion (ROM). It is the most common method of training muscles and has been used extensively for the assessment of muscle performance. The most common method of isotonic muscle performance assessment is the one-repetition maximum lift or the 10-repetition maximum lift. The advantages of this type of exercise and method of muscle performance assessment are:

- It incorporates both concentric and eccentric muscle action
- It strengthens the muscle throughout the ROM
- It is easy to incorporate progressive increases in resistance
- You can exercise multiple joints simultaneously
- It is easily performed in a closed kinetic chain position or gravity dependent position

The main disadvantage of this type of muscle performance is that the weakest point in the ROM limits you when performing the exercise. For example, in the beginning and end of the ROM, you are less able to lift a heavy weight than in the middle of the ROM. Therefore, you are limited to the amount of weight with which you can initiate the lift with and end the lift with when performing an isotonic muscle contraction. Other disadvantages of this type of muscle performance include:

- It is difficult to quantify torque, work, and power
- Stronger muscle groups may compensate for weaker muscle groups, especially during closed-kinetic-chain exercises

Isokinetic Muscle Performance

Isokinetic muscle performance is a dynamic muscle action performed at a fixed speed against a constantly adapting external form of resistance. Most notable forms of external resistance are the isokinetic dynamometers such as the Cybex, KinCom, and Biodex machines. These machines allow for varying speeds of muscle performance and are capable of isolating a joint for specific muscle group action. The advantages of isokinetic exercises and assessment are:

- The accommodating resistance provides maximal resistance throughout the ROM
- The ability to isolate weak muscle groups
- There is an inherent safety mechanism due to the accommodating resistance
- The exercise is velocity controlled
- The ability to quantify torque, work, and power

The disadvantages of this type of exercise are:

- It is primarily performed in an open kinetic chain position
- It is limited to isolated muscle groups
- The exercise is performed through limited cardinal planes of motion
- Some machines do not allow for the eccentric mode of contraction
- The equipment is expensive, space-consuming, and requires a great deal of maintenance.

Current use of isokinetic machinery is primarily seen in the research setting where quantifiable measures of muscle performance are critical and useful in being able to compare data across studies.

BIOMECHANICAL PRINCIPLES OF RESISTANCE EXERCISES

The ability of the musculoskeletal system to function is based upon the following key biomechanical principles:
- Lever—long bones of body
- Fulcrum or pivot point—joints
- Muscle force—muscle contraction
- Resistive force—external source that counters muscle force (eg, gravity, weights, friction)

When a muscle contracts against an external force (eg, dumbbell), the origin and insertion of the muscle are drawn together, thereby pulling on the bone and causing it to rotate about a pivot point or joint. The following terms and definitions are utilized to describe basic biomechanical principles.
- Strength—maximal force a muscle or muscle group generates at a specified velocity
- Acceleration—change in velocity per unit of time
- Power—ability to exert force at high speeds
- Work—product of force times distance
- Torque—measurement of force

As mentioned earlier in this chapter, strength can be measured isometrically, isotonically, or isokinetically depending on the goal in mind. Power, work, and torque can be quantified isokinetically, while acceleration is usually determined by timed functional activities.

BIOMECHANICAL FACTORS THAT AFFECT STRENGTH

With any type of strength training, there is a multitude of factors that affect strength gains. You should consider the following biomechanical factors when prescribing strength training programs and assessing training outcomes:
- Neural control—is dependent on which motor units are recruited and how many. This is why training for sport specificity is so important.
- Muscle cross-sectional area—the greater the size, the greater the strength.
- Arrangement of muscle fibers—angle of pennation (diagonal), the greater the pennation, the greater the strength. For example, the muscle fibers in the adductor magnus muscle are positioned much more diagonally than the muscle fibers in the gracilis muscle. Consequently, the adductor magnus muscle is a much more powerful hip adductor than the gracilis muscle.
- Muscle length—cross-bridge formation is maximized when the muscle is at resting

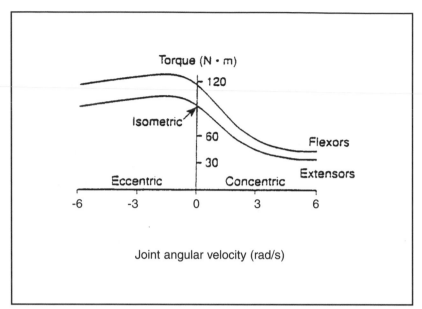

Figure 3-1. Maximal torque capability as a function of joint angular velocity. (Reprinted with permission from: Jorgensen K. Force-velocity relationship in human elbow flexors and extensors. In: Komi PV (ed.). *Biomechanics V-A.* Baltimore: University Park Press; 1976.)

length, which explains why it is easier to lift a weight in the midrange of motion as opposed to the beginning of motion (when the muscle is lengthened) and the end of motion (when the muscle is shortened).
- Joint angle—the higher the torque, the greater tendency for the applied force to rotate the limb about a joint. For example, it is much easier to lift a heavy weight when the weight is held in close to your chest as opposed to straight out in front of you.
- Muscle action velocity—as velocity increases, the ability to generate muscle force decreases. Therefore, keep in mind that less weight will be lifted with high velocity activities such as the power clean, as compared to the dead lift or squat exercises.
- Joint angular velocity—muscle torque varies with joint angular velocity depending on the type of muscle contraction (eg, isometric, isotonic, isokinetic, concentric, eccentric). (Figure 3-1).

The above stated principles of human muscle performance and biomechanical factors that affect strength serve as a basis for strength training prescription. Understanding these principles allows for optimal application of strength training techniques and injury prevention methods.

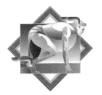

Chapter Four

Techniques of Strength Training

With any activity, it is crucial that the body is prepared with an adequate warm-up and cool-down routine that encompasses a thorough stretching or flexibility program. Different strength training techniques will be discussed in this chapter. An in-depth discussion on stretching and flexibility programs will be addressed in Chapter Fifteen.

WARM-UP AND STRETCHING PERIOD

We recommend approaching the warm-up routine as the foundation for a successful and efficient training session. A brief duration of aerobic activity is necessary to increase the heart rate, respiration rate, blood flow, muscle temperature, and joint viscosity. This enables the muscles and joints to become more resilient, which in turn could possibly decrease the incidence of injury. The warm-up will also allow the body to perform exercises that could possibly allow the lifter to become stronger in a greater range of motion. This would be beneficial to the athletic population. Good examples for a strength training aerobic warm-up are to jump rope, jog, or run through a short obstacle course. Any activity that is engaged in for over 5 to 7 minutes is adequate. You can specify the warm-up to the body parts that will be utilized in the training session. For example, for a lower body workout, a bicycle warm-up may be sufficient. However, if the workout includes the whole body, this should be taken into consideration before beginning the warm-up. The stretching program should immediately follow the aerobic activity. We do suggest that a whole body stretching routine become a regular practice. Although some exercises or lifts may seem primarily specific to a particular body part, they rarely evade usage of the whole body. For example, the power squat may be presumed as strictly a lower body exercise. This is not the case because proper technique utilizes the torso, chest, and shoulder area. The power squat may not work to strengthen the chest and shoulders but if adequate range of motion is not achieved in these areas, effective and efficient form cannot be mastered.

The principles supporting the following exercises have already been discussed in Chapter Three. This chapter will provide background information on the principles of these exercises.

ISOMETRIC EXERCISES

Isometric exercises are primarily used in the rehabilitation arena and are not solely recommended to enhance strength for the healthy athlete. They are, however, beneficial for targeting a specific muscle that may lack strength at a given point in the range of motion or may limit performing a traditional "lift" due to injury. The technique is to statically contract a specific muscle against a fixed resistance and hold the position for more than 6 seconds. The intensity and number of repetitions varies with the need of the athlete. Athletes involved in gymnastics and wrestling are well aware of the need for static strength, but these specific positions should be mastered through the specificity of their workout. Muscle setting is a form of isometric exercise in which the muscles are not contracted against resistance, rather they are contracted maximally by the athletes themselves. An example of this is a "quad set" performed to stimulate quadriceps activity. When the knee is fully extended, the athlete merely tightens the quadriceps muscle. This technique is used primarily during rehabilitation and is worthwhile if the athlete suffers from any form of patellar femoral pain. Examples of applicable isometric exercises are presented in Chapter Seventeen.

ISOTONIC EXERCISES

Combinations of concentric and eccentric muscle contractions are performed with isotonic exercises. The tension developed is less than the resistance load, so the muscle shortens. More force can be generated through the eccentric component as opposed to the concentric muscle contraction.

The simplest and least expensive, yet subjective and inconsistent means of isotonic exercise is the use of a partner. Manual resistance is a form of dynamic resistance in which another person applies opposition to the athlete throughout the range of motion. This method is practical but not always effective for the inexperienced participants. The partner must focus on the athlete performing the contraction in order to make it challenging enough, yet not so much as to cause injury. Resistance machines are also an example of isotonic exercise. Implementation of the machines can save time, especially when performing circuit training. Free-weight equipment is a form of constant resistance in which barbells and dumbbells (DB) are used. They are fairly inexpensive and very versatile. Dumbbells in particular are easy to store, easy to spot, and can be used for numerous upper and lower body exercises. Examples of isotonic exercises are presented in Chapter Seventeen.

PROGRESSIVE RESISTIVE EXERCISES

Progressive resistive exercises (PRE), also known as the DeLorme system, can be implemented as an introductory or preparatory phase for beginning strength trainers. First you need to determine the athlete's 10-repetition maximum (10 RM). The multijoint lifts (ie, bench press, power squat) are best used with this method of strength training. Too much time could be spent assessing each body part if single muscle lifts were incorporated.

The 10 RM can be determined by starting light, having a spotter present, and slowly increasing the weight after each set. A good time to do this is during the orientation of the facility and while educating on proper lifting and spotting techniques. The athlete then performs three sets of 10 repetitions. The routine is as follows:

- First set at 50% of 10 RM
- Second set at 75% of 10 RM
- Third set at 100% of 10 RM

The athlete needs to overload the muscle during the third set, completing the final repetitions with assistance. Once the athlete successfully completes the third set without assistance, the 10RM must be readjusted.

DAILY ADJUSTABLE PROGRESSIVE RESISTANCE EXERCISES (DAPRE)

This method is a taper or pyramid system. The five-repetition maximum (5 RM) is determined, just as with the 10 RM, then the program is as follows:

- First set at 50% 5 RM for 10 repetitions
- Second set at 75% 5 RM for 6 repetitions
- Third set at 100% 5 RM for maximum repetitions
- Fourth set adjusted according to number of repetitions performed in third set

See Table 4-1 for guidelines for adjustment of working weight.

PERIODIZATION

Strength training prescribed in cycles over the course of a training year is known as periodization. The theory of periodization can be very complicated. It is advised to seek the advice of a certified strength and conditioning specialist when questions beyond this text arise. We have attempted to simplify this theory so the different strength training programs can be incorporated during the appropriate cycles. If you are willing to accept the challenge, we suggest acquiring the training schedule and competition calendar for the entire year. This will enable the athletic trainer and the athlete to chart the cycles in the most effective manner.

The macrocycle comprises the overall training period by seasons from preseason and inseason to postseason and off-season. The mesocycle includes two or more cycles (phases) within the macrocycle, such as the introductory, strength, power, and peak phases. The microcycle pertains to the individual weeks of training within the mesocycle. The purpose of this organizational scheme is to decrease the incidence of overtraining and increase optimal strength, peaking at the appropriate time in the season. The time for peaking the athlete will

Table 4-1

GUIDELINES FOR ADJUSTMENT OF WORKING WEIGHT IN THE DAPRE TECHNIQUE

Number of repetitions performed during the third set	Adjusted working weight for the fourth set
0-2	Decrease 5-10 lb
3-4	Decrease 0-5 lb
5-6	Keep the same
7-10	Increase 5-10 lb
> 11	Increase 10-15 lb

Number of repetitions performed during the fourth set	Adjusted working weight for the third set of the following week
0-2	Decrease 5-10 lb
3-4	Keep the same
5-6	Increase 5-10 lb
7-10	Increase 5-15 lb
> 11	Increase 10-20 lb

Reprinted with permission from: National Strength and Conditioning Association. *Essentials of Strength Training and Conditioning.* Champaign, Ill: Human Kinetics; 1994.

depend on the sport activity involved. For example, a basketball or football player needs to be peaked at the beginning of the season because every contest is critical. Whereas a throwing athlete in track and field (this is not to say that these athletes do not emphasize every competition) will want to avoid overtraining or reaching his/her peak too soon due to very high intensity strength programs. This athlete may want to train through multiple contests prior to the conference or qualifying meet. Qualifying meets and conference competitions are usually towards the conclusion of the season in order to meet the demands of the sport. Sports that rely on times (eg, sprinters and swimmers), distances (eg, throwers and jumpers), or heights (eg, vaulters) may complete multiple mesocycles during the season.

Introductory or Preparatory Phase

The introductory or preparatory phase is the period prior to the actual start of the practice season. This phase could last anywhere from 2 to 4 weeks depending on when the athletic trainer is allowed to work with the athlete, when the first competition is scheduled, and when the athlete must peak for performance. It is also when the athlete is introduced or re-introduced to strength training. This is a must for any athlete, beginning or advanced, because it is at this time that the learning curve is overcome and the musculoskeletal system adapts to the loads placed upon it. The emphasis is on the education of lifting and spotting techniques and body preparation for the upcoming months.

The range of repetitions during this phase is 12 to 20 per set. Examples of some effective exercises are super sets, compound sets, complex sets, and pre-exhaustion sets. A super set alternates agonists and antagonists of a joint with minimal to no rest between exercises (eg, bicep curl/tricep pushdown). It can also alternate between upper and lower extremities (eg, bench press/power squat). A compound set uses two different exercises for the same muscle group with minimal to no rest between exercises (eg, lunge/hamstring curl). A complex set uses three to five multijoint exercises with no rest between the exercises (ie, hang clean/front squat/push press). A pre-exhaustion set fatigues an isolated muscle group prior to performing a multi-joint exercise using the same muscle group as its primary mover (eg, DB lying flys/bench press). We suggest you allow 30 seconds of rest for each exercise performed, (eg, during a super set of leg extension and leg curl, allow 1 minute rest prior to the start of the next set.)

Free-weight and body-weight exercises are especially recommended during this phase to emphasize muscle balance and flexibility. This is also a key factor when guiding beginning or younger athletes in perfecting body awareness and coordination. As you will see in Section 6, Sport-Specific Strength Training Programs, back stabilization and torso strength are highly stressed. There is no hurry to advance these two groups into a complicated workout routine. Using solely the body can initiate good stability in the joints, and if done intensely with high volume, provide the athlete with adequate resistance for an excellent strength base. A more advanced but very effective way to increase proprioception, especially for wrestlers, is to perform certain lifts while using a Swiss Ball. For example, while maintaining the bridge position on the ball, the athlete performs DB bench presses. Another idea is to perform DB shoulder exercises while in the sitting position on the ball. This is a great way to combine strength and balance for those athletes who emphasize both areas.

Conditioning at this time is more focused on creating an aerobic base, therefore high volume and low intensity is preferred. Plyometrics are not suggested but if introduced during this time, should be kept to a low volume and low intensity (plyometrics are discussed in Chapter Six). The microcycles within the introductory phase are gradually increased in intensity while the volume is maintained. Again, this phase is the athlete's base, the body's precursor to an efficient and effective season.

Strength Phase

The strength phase progressively increases the intensity while beginning to decrease the volume (discussed in Chapter Five) in both strength training and in conditioning. The repetitions range from eight to 12 repetitions. This permits the athlete to advance to a greater lifting weight, improving not only strength but also joint stability and coordination. The duration of this phase is from 2 to 3 weeks.

Power Phase

During the power phase, the intensity continues to increase while the volume decreases. The exercises and conditioning become more sport specific; the torso stabilization routines and single joint exercises occur less frequently. At this point in the season, the athlete should have excellent core strength and should continue to maintain it. The sets include repetitions from four to eight. This is also a good time to implement plyometrics within the program (ie, superset with an exercise, power squat/box jump, or bench press/medicine ball chest pass), or at the conclusion of the strength training session. The duration of this phase is 2 to 3 weeks.

Peak Phase

The peak phase can also be considered a transition phase. The athlete is transitioning into either the start or the peak portion of the competition season. Remember, as mentioned earlier, some sports indicate a need to peak more than once during a competition season. Emphasis continues on sport specific exercises and conditioning with low volume and high intensity. The programs will shorten in length due to the intensity and rigorous practice/play schedule. The repetitions in this phase can range from one to four for the final set. This practice is addressed in Chapter Eight and is not recommended for those under the age of 16.

The plyometric drills should decrease in quantity (number of sets) and increase in quality (sport specific). For example, if the athlete is engaging in a horizontal type sport (ie, sprinting), the drills should mimic horizontal activity. If the athlete engages in a more vertical sport (eg, jumping), the drills should focus on vertical activity. The peak phase should be no more than 2 weeks, and it should allow adequate rest prior to the desired contest.

In-Season or Maintenance Phase

The in-season or maintenance phase is one that should not be overlooked but not highly emphasized either. Some teams travel more than others, so their time in the weight room may be very limited. The focus here should be on multi-joint exercises in which the programs are performed one to two times a week. This phase continues throughout the season and does not need to cycle within itself. The intensity and volume should continue to be kept relatively low.

Post and Off Season Phase

The post and off-seasons should be a time of active rest. This is a time for recreational sports. This means engaging in activities not specifically related to the competition sport. This is also the opportunity to rehabilitate injuries and merely allow the body to rest. The authors know there are the multi-event/sport and highly motivated athletes who will inquire about continuing with their strength training programs. If this is the case, suggest that those athletes increase the intensity somewhat from the in-season program. Remember that they too need time off at one point during the training year. In Section 6, Sport-Specific Strength Training Programs, golf was given in-season and off-season programs. Often, athletes who participate in tournaments outside their scholastic seasons need more versatility. Therefore, these two programs are basic and can be manipulated by increasing or decreasing the intensity and volume.

CIRCUIT TRAINING

Circuit training is primarily designed to increase muscular endurance, agility, and cardiorespiratory endurance. It involves the performance of a preset series of different exercises. The stations may be organized in a variety of sequences. Focus may be entirely upper or lower body, or one may choose to alternate upper and lower body exercises. The circuit will implement the use of the athlete's body weight primarily, but the use of equipment can add additional resistance and enough variation to decrease staleness. These could vary between cardiovascular pieces and weight room stations, to plyometric supplies and sport specific equipment. The circuit can be adjusted to fit the aerobic or anaerobic needs of the athlete by increasing or decreasing the rest time between stations. The rest may be total rest or active rest depending on the overall goal of the training session. An active rest between stations would involve a slow jog. We recommend a beginner start with six to eight stations, performing each exercise for 15 to 20 seconds with 30 seconds total rest. As the athlete progresses, the stations may increase between 10 and 15, the time of performing the exercises 30 to 45 seconds, and the rest time 15 to 45 seconds of total or active rest. An example of an alternating upper and lower body circuit is as follows. The descriptions of the exercises can be found in the Appendix.

- Squat
- Push-up (regular, incline, decline)
- Walking lunge
- Bench dip
- Step up
- Abdominal crunch
- Jump rope
- Whole body lift

Circuit weight training performed solely in the weight room facility includes a series of lifting exercises performed at 40% to 60% of a one-repetition maximum. This specific type of circuit will reveal modest increases in VO2MAX, but is more apt to increase strength and muscular endurance. We recommend performing each station for 30 seconds, with a 30 to 60 second total rest between. It is important to lift correctly and choose the appropriate load or weight. An example of this type of circuit is as follows, with the descriptions appearing in the Appendix.

- Bench press

- Step up
- Upright row
- Leg extension
- Bicep curl
- Leg curl
- Tricep extension
- Calf raise
- Seated row

COOL-DOWN PERIOD

As the workout shifts from multijoint to single-joint exercises, less energy is needed and the body begins to cool itself. If a conditioning, plyometric, or sport-specific workout is not to follow the outlined strength training program, then a brief all-body stretch will be adequate for the session's cool down. However, if more training is expected, the body should be kept warm and moving until completion of the last period of training. When the training session is concluded, a routine of low-intensity activity (eg, slow jog) and light stretching is recommended to improve recovery from the workout.

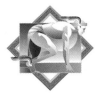

Chapter Five

Strength Training Prescription

Now with a basic understanding of the principles behind human muscle performance and the various strength training techniques, we can focus on the four domains involved in prescribing strength training programs.

These domains are critical to the effectiveness of the strength program because all four areas intertwine with each workout. Intensity is not only a mindset, but also a quantitative figure of just how much weight is being moved in a given repetition. Volume encompasses the entire set and multiplies the number of repetitions with the intensity. Frequency helps to limit detraining or overtraining. Without recovery, there might be a higher incidence of injury with little strength gains.

INTENSITY

Intensity in strength training is the amount of weight one lifts per repetition. This can range from one's own body weight to the use of various dumbbell and barbell weights. We suggest when beginning with young and beginning strength trainers, you emphasize body weight exercises. Examples and suggestions are discussed in Chapter Eight.

Generalizing the weights for all of your athletes may lead to embarrassment for the beginner, lack of positive results for the advanced, and may increase the possibility of injury. Therefore, a repetition maximum (RM) must first be established for every athlete for each major lift. We do not suggest testing the single-joint exercises. This practice is more effective and suggested with the multijoint lifts (ie, bench press and power clean). To save time and frustration on your part, it is imperative that you refer to the following factors that may influence initial accuracy of maximum testing.

- Conditioning: Are the athletes well conditioned or have they ever conditioned?
- Familiarity: Are they comfortable with the exercise, with the equipment, with their spotter, with you?
- Coaching: Have they been instructed in strength training and spotting techniques?
- Fatigue: Have they just completed a strenuous workout? Have they prefatigued a specific muscle group?

- Recovery times between trials: Are they allowing a full recovery between sets?
- Type of weight equipment used: Are they accustomed to barbells as opposed to dumbells? Are they accustomed to free weights as opposed to machines?
- Personal motivation: Is this being forced or do they want to excel in this area?

It is a good idea to start beginners with a 10 repetition maximum (10 RM) test. After a proper warm-up/stretching and instruction of strength training and spotting techniques, begin with a light to moderate weight. For some, it may be a stripped barbell. If the barbell is too heavy, the use of dumbbells is appropriate. Each and every lift can be modified to meet the needs of the young, old ,and physically challenged. Remember to initialize your beginners with body weight and dumbbell exercises so their transition into the more advanced strength training techniques will pose little complication.

If the athlete has completed a set of 10 repetitions and found it to be less than challenging, continue to add 5 to 15 lbs until the athlete is able to only complete the final repetition with assistance. For the beginner, this will be a long process. It may take you and the athlete four or five sets to determine the 10 RM. Remember to allow full recovery between sets to eliminate fatigue as a factor. Patience is crucial; take the time to give them valuable instruction and guidance along the way. The learning curve will advance the beginners much faster early on in the program. Modification during observation and instruction will ensure the athlete is progressing in a safe, efficient, and effective manner.

The 10RM will be an estimated 72.5% of the potential 1 RM. With this percentage, and knowing what mesocycle the athlete is in, you can determine the relative intensity for each set. As the athlete progresses from the introductory to peak phase, the intensity increases. The volume (discussed in the next section) will decrease as intensity increases; therefore, the volume will determine how the percentages (of 1 RM) are spaced within the set.

As the athletes progress in chronological age and experience, the 10 RM can be modified to a 5 RM, 3 RM, or even 1 RM for evaluation purposes. We do not suggest that anyone under the age of 16 engage in the 1 RM. This is to protect the athlete from the possibility of injury, such as damaging the growth plates. Unless the athlete is a competitive power or Olympic lifter, the 1 RM is not critical for continued strength gains (this is discussed in more detail in Chapter Eight). The working relative intensity can still be computed with a 3 RM or 5 RM, or if you are working with an endurance athlete, keep the 10 RM for evaluation purposes. Re-emphasize to the athlete the importance of proper technique both by the lifter and spotter and to only perform the repetition maximum tests under skilled professionals' supervision.

VOLUME

The total workload during a series of sets is considered the volume (product of total amount of weight and total number of repetitions). The volume, like intensity, of training will depend entirely on the mesocycle or phase at which the athlete is currently working. As the repetitions decrease with the increasing weight of each set (intensity), the volume proportionally decreases. The introductory phase will begin with light to moderate weight and high repetitions. The peak phase will emphasize heavy weight and low repetitions. A higher number of repetitions is used for the body's introduction to strength training, endurance or circuit training. The implementation of lower repetitions progresses for the maximal strength and power gains.

Now that we have shown how intensity and volume are related, we can determine and space the percentages between the first and final sets. You can use the following information as a guideline. The first (or warm-up) set will always start with 50% to 60% of the 1RM. So, if the last set of the exercise is:

- Ten to 15 repetitions, use 72.5% to 70% of the 1RM respectively for the subsequent sets.
- Six to eight repetitions, use 82.5% to 77.5% of the 1RM respectively for the subsequent sets.
- Two to four repetitions, use 87.5% to 92.5% of the 1RM respectively for the subsequent sets.

For example, a bench press workout in which the athlete has to perform one set of eight repetitions and three sets of six repetitions may look like eight repetitions at 50% of 1 RM, six repetitions at 60%, six repetitions at 72.5%, and the final six repetitions at 82.5%. It is important to remember that each microcycle (week) within the mesocycle (phase) will need to be evaluated and modified to accommodate the changing weights, sets, and repetitions.

FREQUENCY

The frequency is the number of training sessions in a specific duration of time. This number is specific to each athlete. The season of year is probably the most important determining factor of frequency. You would not want an athlete training four to five times a week in the in-season or post-season, just as you would not want the athlete to train just one to two times in the preseason. Both scenarios would produce less than desirable effects. The health status, training, and experience level are also indicators of how many times the athlete will train in a 1-week period. Athletes who have maintained an adequate level of strength and fitness should recover faster than the beginner and thus be able to complete more training sessions in a given period of time.

The frequency of the beginner should be kept to a minimum. It is appropriate to alternate strength training days. As the lifter advances, it is not unusual for him/her to train four or five, even six sessions per week. Again, this depends on the level and goal of the athlete.

Another factor that could increase or decrease the frequency is the type of exercises and how they are performed. Eccentric and multijoint exercises will require more recovery than single-joint exercises. This is due to the eccentric contraction causing more strain as it lengthens the muscle and the high energy being expended with the use of multiple muscles. To summarize these three sections in one simple thought, the lower the volume (less repetitions), the higher the intensity (more weight), the lower the frequency (fewer training sessions).

RECOVERY

The recovery period between sets, exercises, and training sessions is as critical as the program itself. The amount of rest is purely dependent upon the energy source being utilized and depleted, thus dependent upon the training goal of each specific athlete.

It is advised that the athlete permit a muscle group 48 hours to recover. If a muscle group is used as a primary mover during the first session, using it as a secondary mover the next session is not discouraged, nor is it encouraged. This is usually unavoidable with the athlete due to implementing power and Olympic lifts. The Olympic lifts are performed during a lower body training session; however, in order to effectively and efficiently complete the lift, smaller muscle groups used during the previous session will have to be utilized.

Circuit training, for example, incorporates strength and aerobic endurance components. When the exercise involves the body as resistance, low weight, or a single joint, a 1:1 work to rest ratio is suggested. For example, if the exercise requires 20 seconds to complete, the rest for that set is 20 seconds. Circuit training should not be emphasized during the entire mesocycle but be introduced to break the monotony, confuse the muscles, and allow them to adapt. Transitioning from one mesocycle to another, choosing one or two training sessions, is another time to incorporate circuit training.

Muscle endurance training emphasizes rest periods of 30 to 60 seconds between sets. This works well for athletes involved in endurance sports or who must produce quick boosts of power over a long period of time (eg, basketball).

For absolute strength, a complete recovery (approximately 2.5 to 3 minutes) between sets is required. This will replenish phosphagen (ATP and phosphocreatine) stores, which can be depleted within 15 seconds of intense lifting. This is practiced during the peak phase, as the athlete culminates the previous training weeks and begins to transition into the competition season. The throwing events in track and field truly benefit from this because of their demand for absolute power. The athlete who can generate the most force the quickest will throw the farthest.

In conclusion, it is the authors' suggestion that athletic trainers arrange a time with the athlete or team to evaluate the season. As discussed in Chapter Four, break the macrocycle (training year) into mesocycles (phases), beginning with the introductory, and transitioning into the strength, power, and peak phases. The final peak phase will transition the athlete into the competition season. Now, break the mesocycles into microcycles and determine the intensity and volume of each multijoint lift. The sport specific programs in Chapter Eighteen provide suggestions. Once the athlete has completed the orientation and you have evaluated his/her base strength for the multilifts, he or she is ready to begin the strength training program. Remember the key to an effective and efficient program is to continue to instruct, observe, and evaluate your athletes.

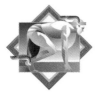 Chapter Six

Plyometrics

Two of an athletes' most desired physical strategies over the opponent are that of strength and speed. Maximizing the two into one is the development of power. Plyometrics are training drills that bridge that gap between strength and speed.

It does not matter in what sport the athlete is engaged; power will always be advantageous. The sports that do not transfer well are those of repetition, such as cycling. However, swimming, which is also a repetition sport, can benefit from drills to increase power during the wall turn.

PRINCIPLES

What makes plyometrics work as a training tool is the use of potential energy, kinetic energy, and the myotatic reflex (also know as the stretch reflex). Potential energy is that which is stored in the muscles due to the force of gravity. The myotatic reflex senses eccentric contractions through the muscle spindles, causing the same muscle to contract along with the synergist muscles, while simultaneously inhibiting the antagonist muscles by way of the Golgi tendon organ. Kinetic energy converts the potential energy into maximal force through a countermovement. To summarize this in a more practical application, as the athlete steps down from an elevated surface, kinetic energy is stored. The transition between landing and jumping uses the myotatic reflex. How much tension is exerted and how high he/she will jump depends on the kinetic energy.

PHASES

Generally, the phases of plyometrics are the downward phase, the countermovement, and the upward phase. The downward phase is the stepping or jumping down from an apparatus. It can also occur while approaching a landing from a jump. This phase requires the least amount of effort but is still significant for potential energy, because maximal tension develops when active muscles are stretched quickly. The countermovement, or amortization phase, is most critical. This phase begins as the athlete impacts the surface and ends when he/she initiates acceleration. The idea is to make this time on the ground as short as possible. The muscle exerts more force the faster it is forced to lengthen (a pause would dissipate rather than use this stored energy). The analogy of a check mark is very useful when trying to emphasize this phase. The point of the check mark is very sharp. This point is the amortization phase, the time spent on the ground. Therefore, in order to keep this point sharp, the athlete must rapidly counter from an eccentric to concentric contraction. The upward acceleration phase is the explosive concentric contraction. The ability to move quickly is not as effective if you are unable to contract completely and rebound efficiently. The tension exerted increases as you increase your elastic strength, your ability to maximally utilize the kinetic energy in the muscle.

PLYOMETRIC PRESCRIPTION

Prior to implementing a plyometric program, it is highly recommended that the athlete complete an extensive introductory strength training phase. This will strengthen the muscles adequately to increase the effectiveness of the training, while perhaps decreasing the incidence of injury.

To maximize the training, because quality is more important than quantity, it is suggested that the athlete try to perform lower extremity plyometric drills on predominantly upper body strength training days. Also, they are best to do before the conditioning session and on speed training days. It would be counterproductive to perform drills that emphasize power then condition for endurance. The same is suggested for upper extremity plyometric drills. Try to place them on the predominantly lower body strength training days.

It will be necessary to warm-up specific to the plyometric training session. For the upper extremity session, a set of push-ups with an adequate stretch will be sufficient. For the lower extremity session, a brief duration of aerobic activity is necessary to increase the heart rate, respiration rate, blood flow, muscle temperature, and joint viscosity. This enables the muscles and joints to become more resilient, which in turn could possibly decrease the incidence of injury. Good examples are jump rope, slow jog, or running a short obstacle course. Any activity that is engaged for over 5 to 7 minutes is adequate.

The frequency of plyometric training sessions should be one to three times per week depending on the strength of the athlete and where in the macrocycle (training year) he or she is currently working. If it is early, for example during the strength phase, then once a week is sufficient. As the athlete transitions into the power and peak phases, two times a week on the days suggested above is recommended. The only time three training sessions should be implemented is for the athlete who is advanced in strength and plyometric training and has the ability to train through and peak multiple times during the season. Track and field is an example of a sport that selects specific competitions to peak as opposed to each contest being critical to the postseason rankings.

The volume is also dependent upon the athlete, the type of drills, and the phase. You must advance the athlete in plyometric training, just as you do in strength training. For beginners or those in the strength phase, it is advised to keep the contacts between 70 and 100. Each time the foot or feet land on the ground is considered a contact. Intermediate athletes or those in the power phase can progress to between 100 and 120. Advanced and peak phase athletes should complete no more than 140 contacts. Remember to keep in mind that quality is the key and not quantity. If the drills are not being performed efficiently and effectively, then the training session should be discontinued until adequate rest and recovery can be obtained. Full recovery is a must between drills and training sessions. The next set in a session should not be executed until the athlete has regained normal breathing. Like strength training, a period of 48 hours is recommended to recover between sessions.

Once again, the intensity will depend on the athlete. Beginners should start their program with two feet landings without obstacles. As the athlete progresses, he/she may implement one-foot landings and drills that incorporate cones or hurdles. As the intensity (level of drill) increases, the volume (number of repetitions) should decrease.

Choosing the appropriate drills should be indicative of the sport involved. Is the sport vertical (high jumper) or horizontal (sprinter)? Does the athlete rely on explosive power (shot putter) versus reactive power (triple jumper)? Vertical drills are those that require the athlete to jump in a vertical manner; the bounding drills are an example of a horizontal drill. Explosive drills are those such as depth jumps; and reactive drills are the repetitive jumping drills. Analyze each drill to ensure that the time spent is worthwhile.

When working with young people, only low intensity drills should be used. Examples include jump rope, hops, and jumps. They should not engage in high intensity drills such as bounding and box jumps until their personal physician has determined them of adequate physical maturity (eg, Tanner scale of 5).

Consider the following prior to implementing a plyometric program:

* Adequate strength base.
* Physical maturity of athlete.
* Physical size of athlete; decrease intensity when working with larger (>90 kgs) athletes.
* Mesocycle, recommended during the power and peak phases.
* Jumping surface, too soft will absorb kinetic energy.
* Shoes should have good ankle support and non-slip sole.
* Boxes should be sturdy, appropriate height, and have a non-slip surface.
* Hurdles and cones should be of good quality.
* Know the specifics of the sport, vertical versus horizontal and explosive versus reactive.
* Adequate rest between drills, and recovery between sessions.
* Adequate supervision, a must for every training session to ensure fatigue does not affect training session and increase incidence of injury.

Within the sport specific-programs in Chapter Eighteen, there are suggestions for upper and lower extremity plyometric drills and when to incorporate them into the program. The supplemental programs in Chapter Seventeen describe each drill in detail. The numbers on the specific sport programs correspond to the numbers on the descriptions in Chapter Seventeen.

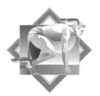

Chapter Seven

Special Populations

Prepubescent and Adolescent Age Athletes

If the children are the future, why not educate them early on the benefits of exercise and strength training? Developing strong habits as young people will produce adults with solid foundations of health. It is no secret that today more adults are overweight, sedentary, and in danger of dying younger due to diseases that might have been prevented with exercise and a healthier diet. It is painful to see physical education programs being dropped from school curriculums across the nation. The idea that administrations and parents still embrace the concerns of yesterday is disturbing. The following are some of the benefits that young people experience when engaging in activities such as strength training:

- Increase muscle strength and endurance
- Increase muscle balance, coordination, and motor skills
- Increase self-confidence, discipline, and respect
- Provide socialization and opportunities for building leadership skills
- Help control weight and reduce fat
- Prevent or delay the development of high blood pressure
- According to The Center for Disease Control and Prevention, may help reduce blood pressure in some adolescents with hypertension
- And most encouraging, may increase bone mass.

Every one of these benefits, or even just one, is reason enough to implement a strength training program for young people. However, there does still exist both emotional and medical concerns with strength training for prepubescent and adolescent age athletes. The most often cited arguments against strength training for this group are:

1. They are incapable of making significant strength gains due to inadequate levels of androgens.

2. Strength training is dangerous and has an increased risk of injury.

Sewall and Micheli (1984) examined 18 prepubescent children of both genders. The intervention group participated in a progressive resistive exercise strength training program three times a week for 9 weeks. The intervention group showed a mean increase in strength of 42.9%, control 9.5%. Numerous studies have since been completed to support the idea that the strengths gained in the prepubescent and adolescent age groups are due to the adaptations of the neurological and muscular systems. The muscle fibers and groups merely learn to coordinate and they contract more efficiently; therefore, they are able to move with increased force.

Aside from acute injuries, which may or may not be avoidable, 30% to 50% of all pediatric sports injuries are due to overuse. Overuse occurs in any age group when training has been progressed too rapidly and not enough rest and recovery has been allocated. Under the direct supervision of a certified professional, this factor should be 100% avoidable. There are cases of sport-specific related injuries. Too many times, young athletes are enrolled in sports camps for multiple consecutive days when they are not physically or mentally, ready to participate. Again, if you stress even an adult who is accustomed to a moderate routine and abruptly increase that activity, there is a chance that an overuse injury will occur. So, in order to help prevent overuse injuries, it is highly suggested that the sport activity be monitored with the same intensity as the strength training program. The following criteria are recommended for implementing a strength training program for a prepubescent or adolescent athlete:

- Witness the enthusiasm of the athlete to participate
- Insist a physician has given each participant a thorough physical examination prior to exercise training and clearance for participation
- Suggest the physician evaluate and correct for the possibility of anorexia or amenorrhea
- Keep signed legal documents (eg, parent's awareness of risk and medical questionnaire) on file
- Determine maturity and ability to listen and follow directions; a 10-year-old may be more successful than a 12-year-old
- Advocate strength training as a part of a whole body wellness plan, including flexibility, nutrition, and cardiovascular fitness. For example, not all young people consume the recommended calcium intake of 1200 to 1500 mg/d
- Educate how to perform and why we need a proper warm-up and cool down.
- Instruct on proper strength training techniques
- Progress training from two to no more than three sessions a week
- Keep training sessions between 30 and 60 minutes for attention span and interest.

The best method of strength training for the young athlete is to incorporate exercises that utilize his/her own body weight. This includes, but is not limited to, sit-ups, push-ups, dips, pull-ups, squats, and lunges. In fact, a body weight exercise can be implemented for every body part and examples will be provided at the end of this section. Emphasis on the postural musculature is critical and can be accomplished by exercising through bilateral and unilateral movements. This developed stability in the torso may aid in coordination of activity and decrease the incidence of injury, notably to the low back region.

Alternating training sessions of 30 minutes three times a week is ample. Obviously, attention span and level of athleticism will determine this. We as athletic trainers can better hold the athlete's attention through circuit training, use of different equipment, or integrating a partner or group. Furthermore, the benefit of a circuit enables adequate recovery when changing the sequence of body parts. Emphasis should be on using the body as resistance or low weight resistance for 10 to 20 repetitions. Rather than continuing to increase the weight lifted, increase the number of repetitions performed. For example, if an athlete can perform the dumbbell bench press easily 12 to 15 repetitions with 5 pounds, increase the set to 20 repetitions using the same 5 pounds. Once this is mastered, increase the athlete to 7.5 pounds for 12 to 15 repetitions and so on.

Dumbbells are excellent for strength enhancement because they emphasize coordination, bilateral muscle balance, and full range of motion. Exercises involving overhead lifting are often a cause of injury due to inadequate trunk and shoulder strength or stability, and should be avoided until the athlete has developed this strength and stability.

Maximal lifting is contraindicated for prepubescent and adolescent athletes due to their underdeveloped musculotendinous junctions and growth plates. The United States Weight and Power Lifting Federations recommend the athlete be 14 years of age. The National Strength and Conditioning Association has suggested we assess physical maturity on an individual basis and never permit participants under the age of 16 to engage in maximal lifting. A widely accepted guideline is that based on physical maturation. Once the athlete reaches a Tanner stage 5 in development, his/her maximum velocity height growth period has been passed. Therefore, the opportunity for injury is minimal in the areas of growth plates. The mean age of reaching Tanner stage 5 is 15 years in both genders. Again, individualism is the key to a safe and productive strength training program. The following are examples of beginning body weight programs:

1. Jump rope 2 minutes (see Section 6 for details):
   - Feet together x 30 sec.
   - Single leg (alternating right then left) x 30 sec.
   - Double right/double left etc. x 30 sec.
   - Single right only x 15 sec.
   - Single left only x 15 sec.
   - Stretch 10 minutes (see Chapter Fifteen)
   - Abdominal crunches 3 x 30 seconds (continuing repetitions), rest 60 seconds between sets back extensions on floor 4 x 15 seconds (continuing repetitions), rest 30 seconds between sets
   - Squats 4 x 30 seconds (continuing repetitions), rest 1 minute between each set
   - Walking lunges, 30 paces per leg, no rest.
   - Standing single heel raises 3 x 15 seconds (continuing repetitions) right then left, no rest, standing/seated toe taps 3 x 15 seconds (continuing repetitions) right then left, no rest
   - Stretch 5 minutes.

2. Jog 5 minutes (see Section 6 for details).
   - Stretch 10 minutes
   - Back stabilization exercises (see Section 6)
   - Hip routine (see Section 6)
   - Incline pull-ups 2 x 20 seconds, rest 40 seconds between each set
   - Push-ups 4 x 30 seconds, rest 30 seconds between each set
   - Tennis ball squeezes 3 x 15 seconds (continuing repetitions) right then left, no rest

- Bench dips 4 x 30 seconds, rest 1 minute between each set
- Crab crawls 3 x 30 seconds, rest 30 seconds between each set (supine, hands and feet on ground and move forward)
- Bear walks 3 x 15 seconds, rest 30 seconds between each set (prone, hands and feet on ground and move forward)
- Stretch 5 minutes.

Partner exercises may include:

- Relay races
- Wheel barrow walks
- Medicine ball tosses (see Section 6)
- Medicine ball abdominal (see Section 6).

3. Example of weight room programs (see Section 6 for details)

Day 1 and 3:

- Bike/jog/jump rope 5 minutes
- Stretch 10 minutes
- Rotator cuff warm up
- Push-ups
- Dumbbell (DB) lying flys
- DB/barbell bench press
- DB front raise (light)
- DB upright row
- Bench dips/tricep pushdown
- DB hammer curls/bicep curls
- Abdominal curls
- Stretch 5 minutes.

Day 2:

- Bike/jog/jump rope 5 minutes
- Stretch 10 minutes
- Hip routine (see Section 6)
- Back stabilization (see Section 6)
- DB/barbell squats
- DB lunges
- DB calf raises
- DB bentover row
- Lateral pulldown
- Stretch 5 minutes.

WOMEN

When it comes to strength training, there are anatomical differences between men and women that result in greater amounts of muscle tissue in men as compared to women. The primary anatomical differences between men and women are as follows:

1. Body height, with men typically being taller than women
2. Body weight, with men typically weighing more than women
3. Muscle fiber size, which is greater in men due to higher levels of testosterone
4. Hip width : shoulder width ratios, which are greater in women due to increased pelvic width in women and decreased shoulder width as compared to men
5. Percent body fat, which is greater in women than men.

Women average about two-thirds the strength of men. Female upper body strength is said to be about 30% to 50% of male upper body strength. When strength comparisons are made relative to lean body mass, men and women are more comparable, however differences are still present. Although there are anatomical differences between men and women, strength training adaptations are similar for both men and women, except for the extent of increase in muscle fiber size. When strength is assessed according to the cross-sectional area of a muscle, the ability to generate force is independent of gender. Although anatomical differences are present, there is no reason why women should be kept from engaging in strength training activities. In fact, women should be encouraged to strength train, especially when the benefits of strength training and aging are considered.

SENIORS

It is well known that after puberty, strength reaches its peak potential. It maintains a plateau until about the age of 50 years, after which strength declines, with a more rapid decline seen after the age of 60 years. This is due to the following factors:

1. More sedentary lifestyle
2. Decreased activity in neuromuscular system
    a. Loss of functional motor units
    b. Slower nerve conduction velocity
    c. Decreased endocrine activity
3. Decreased muscle mass
    a. Decreased number of muscle fibers
    b. Decreased muscle fiber size
    c. Preferential loss of fast-twitch muscle fibers
    d. Increased fat and connective tissue
4. Decreased intramuscular blood flow
5. Changes in contractile proteins and protein metabolism.

Although these changes cannot be reversed, the rate of change can be slowed with strength training in the elderly. It is possible for older participants to see hypertrophy changes and other physiological adaptations with strength training exercises.

We recommend that strength training programs be highly supervised during the introduction of a strength training program to ensure proper technique and progression.

Strength gains in an older population are attributed to the utilization of sufficient training intensity and duration. Increases in strength may range from 10% to 175%. Increases in cross-sectional area may range from 5% to 15%. Most of the training programs that resulted in these increases consisted of both concentric and eccentric muscle contractions performed three times a week for approximately 12 weeks. Training intensities ranged from 65% to 80% of a one-repetition maximum lift for each exercise. Some older individuals may even be involved in organized sports or lifetime activities. The strength training programs outlined in Section 6 can also apply to this population. Just remember that with any training program; always obtain physician clearance prior to exercise prescription in a senior population. Also, be certain to adapt strength training exercises to meet the needs of individual athletes. This is especially important in the older population due to pathological considerations such as musculoskeletal injuries, osteoarthritis conditions, joint replacements, diabetes, cardiovascular disease, and medication contraindications.

HUMAN IMMUNODEFICIENCY VIRUS/ACQUIRED IMMUNODEFICIENCY SYNDROME

Since the discovery of the human immunodeficiency virus (HIV) and acquired immunodeficiency syndrome (AIDS), a number of issues in the athletic arena have been addressed. Two major concerns are the transmission of the virus and disease, and whether those infected with HIV and AIDS should participate in physical activity.

First, the modes of assumed transmission we will focus on are through blood, sweat, saliva, and tears. It was discovered very early that blood was a major transportation system for the virus and disease. Pertinent to athletics may be the possibilities that participants may share needles and syringes with someone who is infected, and that there is a chance that during contact or collision sport activity, and the care of said sports, someone who is infected may come in contact with someone who is not infected.

According to the Centers for Disease Control and Prevention, there has been only one reported case of HIV transmission from a healthcare worker to a patient. Since then they have investigated more than 22,000 patients of HIV-infected surgeons, physicians, and dentists. No additional infections were found.

A health care worker has a higher chance of contracting the Hepatitis B virus than HIV or AIDS. There are approximately 9,000 reported cases of contracted Hepatitis B by health care workers each year. There are to date approximately 56 reported cases of HIV contracted through occupational health care.

There is one report in Italy of an athlete transmitting HIV to another player, however this case is undocumented. Although HIV has been found in sweat, saliva, and tears, there has never been a case of transmission by these means. So, it appears that the likelihood of an athlete contracting HIV or AIDS during participation in a sport is rare. Chances are, you have or will have an athlete that has been infected with HIV and may or may not know it at the time. Confidentiality, and the fact that some cases go undetected for many years prevents us from knowing exactly who is and is not infected. Certified Athletic Trainers and those who assist with wound care should continue to follow the guidelines of universal precautions regardless of the patient.

Specialists in AIDS and HIV research and treatment have claimed for a number of years that HIV-positive people who are asymptomatic and do not have an active infection may participate in moderate to high levels of physical activity. Obviously, each person and case should be evaluated on an individual basis. The effects of exercise may be even more advantageous for those infected. Benefits such as increasing cardiovascular fitness, reducing levels of stress and depression, and that of building lean muscle mass are especially desirable for infected individuals. The additional muscle mass may provide a buffer against the eventual wasting that will occur as the disease progresses.

If by chance we are made aware of an infected athlete, it is very important to keep his/her status confidential. This may help in preventing unnecessary discrimination from other participants. We may also provide some helpful recommendations. Since HIV/AIDS patients have an increased resting metabolic rate, it would be worthwhile to increase their intake of calories. While doing this, education in nutrition and vitamin supplementation should also be emphasized. Often appetite is decreased, therefore the addition of certain weight gain products that are on the market may help along the way.

It seems that the implementation of education in this area would relieve many concerns revolving around the participation of HIV/AIDS athletes. We recommend contacting your local organizations for up-to-date information on the disease. Educate your administrators, parents, athletes, and coworkers on the advantages of encouraging those infected to participate in a healthy exercise program.

DIABETICS

The types and mechanisms of diabetes mellitus are discussed in detail in Chapter Twelve. Our focus in this section is on strength training techniques as they apply to the diabetic individual, whereas endurance training recommendation, are presented in Chapter Twelve.

Strength training for the diabetic athlete should be encouraged for many of the same beneficial reasons that apply to normal, healthy individuals. With careful preparticipation screening and training supervision, resistance training in the diabetic athlete can result in increased muscular strength and endurance, improved insulin sensitivity and glucose tolerance, enhanced body composition, improved flexibility, and decreased risk factors associated with cardiovascular disease. Careful preparticipation screening is necessary to identify those individuals at risk for strength training exercises due to microvascular or neurological compromise, or cardiovascular disease.

As with intense endurance training, some diabetics should avoid intense strength training. For example, individuals who have cardiovascular complications as a result of disease progression should avoid intense strength training exercises. Intensive strength training may produce a short-term hyperglycemic effect during or immediately after the training session. A hypoglycemic response is then expected many hours after exercise in response to the restoration of muscle gylcogen. Additionally, it is advised that diabetics eliminate exhaustive exercise, and limit isometric exercise performance. Unless proper breathing techniques are utilized isometric exercises can lead to increased blood pressure and excessive demands on the cardiovascular system. Breathing techniques during lifting should consist of exhalation during the upward lift and inhalation during the downward lift. It is especially important that they do not hold their breath.

In order to control the glycemic responses, the diabetic athlete should monitor his/her blood glucose levels before, during, and after strength training. Recommendations for carbohydrate consumption and insulin dosages are presented in Chapter Twelve. We also recommend that training programs are introduced gradually and monitored carefully so that adaptations can be made as needed.

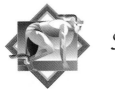

Section 3

Endurance Training

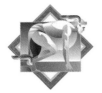

Chapter Eight

Principles of Cardiorespiratory Performance

For any athlete, the importance of cardiorespiratory function cannot be overlooked. The cardiorespiratory system is responsible for delivering adequate amounts of oxygen to the working muscles and is essential in removing the byproducts of exercise. The transport and exchange of oxygen (O_2) and carbon dioxide (CO_2) is of utmost importance in maintaining homeostasis during exercise. The circulatory system is also important in transporting the necessary energy sources for muscle function. In addition, body temperature is regulated by the circulatory system. This chapter will focus on the basic components and function of the circulatory and respiratory systems, as well as describe the pertinent energy systems for muscle function. The following chapters will incorporate these basic concepts and identify techniques of endurance training. Examples will be provided for prescribing endurance training in normal individuals, active individuals, and special populations.

CIRCULATORY SYSTEM

The heart is considered a muscular pump with four chambers and four one-way valves. The myocardium is the middle muscular layer of the heart that is responsible for chamber contraction and movement of blood through the heart to the major vessels, where it is dispensed to the rest of the body. Unlike skeletal muscle, the myocardium is made up of intercalated discs that permit transmission of electrical impulses and allow for the inherent rhythmicity that maintains continuous heart function. The myocardium is similar to skeletal muscle in that it is striated and contains actin and myosin. This allows the heart to contract using the sliding filament theory. The myocardium is a highly aerobic muscle containing a large number of mitochondria and an extensive blood supply.

The cardiac cycle is the contraction and relaxation phase of the heart. Systole is known as the contraction phase, while diastole is known as the relaxation phase. Both the atria and ventricles contract and relax. When the atria is in systole, the ventricles are in diastole. At rest, the heart beats, or contracts and relaxes, at 75 beats per minute. During exercise, an elevated heart rate results in less time spent in diastole.

Blood pressure is the force exerted by blood against the arterial walls. This is determined by how much blood is pumped and by the amount of resistance to blood flow. Systolic blood pressure is produced when the ventricles contract; diastolic blood pressure occurs during ventricular relaxation. Normal blood pressure for males is 120/80 mmHg, whereas normal blood pressure for females is 110/70 mmHg. During exercise, systolic blood pressure increases to pump the increased blood volume to the working muscles. Elevated systolic blood pressure is considered normal up to 220 mmHg.

Cardiac output is a function of stroke volume (SV) and heart rate (HR). The SV represents the amount of blood pumped per heart beat, and HR is equal to the number of beats per minute. Normal cardiac output at rest for males is 5.00 l/min, and normal cardiac output at rest for females is 4.50 l/min. During exercise, cardiac output increases to 18.0 to 34.2 l/min. Initially this increase is due to an increase in both SV and HR. SV can increase as much as 64% with exercise. As work rate increases, the increase in cardiac output is due primarily to a continued HR increase. HR may increase up to 180 to 200 beats/min. with intense exercise. This is necessary in order to meet the demands of increased gas exchange and energy usage.

RESPIRATORY SYSTEM

Pulmonary respiration involves the lungs, which provide a means of gas exchange between the environment and the body. It occurs through the processes of ventilation and diffusion. Ventilation is the process of moving air into and out of the lungs. Diffusion is the movement of molecules from high concentration to low concentration and occurs in the alveoli of the lungs. Diffusion is controlled by the partial pressures of O_2 and CO_2. During inspiration, the diaphragm contracts and lowers, expanding the thoracic cavity. The ribs are also lifted outward, thereby reducing intrapleural pressure resulting in lung expansion. During expiration, the diaphragm and ribs passively relax, forcing air out of the lungs.

Pulmonary ventilation is the movement of gas in and out of the lungs and is based upon the frequency of breaths and tidal volume. Tidal volume is the amount of gas ventilated per minute at rest. Pulmonary capacity takes into account the tidal volume, inspiratory and expiratory reserve volumes, vital capacity, and residual volume. The inspiratory reserve volume is the volume of gas inspired after normal tidal inspiration. The expiratory reserve volume is the volume of gas expired after normal tidal expiration. The inspiratory and expiratory reserve volumes are utilized during exercise to allow for increased O_2 and CO_2 exchange.

Vital capacity (VC) is the maximum amount of gas expired after maximum inspiration. It is the voluntary amount of maximal inhalation and exhalation. The residual volume (RV) is the gas that remains in the lungs after maximum expiration. It is this amount of gas that prevents the lungs from completely deflating. Total lung capacity is the sum of the VC and RV. It represents the maximum amount of air we can voluntarily move in and out of our lungs, plus the gas reserve that remains in the lungs.

Cellular respiration involves gas exchange in the tissues. Hemoglobin is a blood protein that binds to O_2 in the blood for transport and becomes oxyhemoglobin. Dissociation of oxygen from hemoglobin occurs at the tissues and is dependent on the partial pressure of O_2 and hemoglobin saturation. With an increased partial pressure of O_2, we see formation of oxyhemoglobin, whereas with a decreased partial pressure of O_2, we see unloading of O_2 from hemoglobin, also known as deoxyhemoglobin.

The exchange of O_2 and CO_2 in the tissues occurs in the capillaries. The arterio-venous oxygen difference (a-v O_2 diff) represents the amount of oxygen being extracted by the tissue cells. Myoglobin is a blood protein that binds to O_2 in the muscles. There are large quantities of myoglobin in slow-twitch muscle fibers to accommodate their aerobic characteristics. There is less myoglobin in fast-twitch muscle fibers that are primarily anaerobic in nature. Carbon dioxide is transported three different ways: dissolved in the blood (10%), bound to hemoglobin (carbaminohemoglobin) (20%), or as bicarbonate (HCO_3) (70%). It is this tissue exchange of O_2 and CO_2 that ultimately provides an optimal environment for energy metabolism and exercise function.

Acid-base balance control is important in maintaining homeostasis during pulmonary ventilation. It is dictated by hydrogen ion concentration and can be controlled by the formation of HCO_3. Substances that release hydrogen are considered acids, and substances that combine with hydrogen are labeled bases. Acid-base balance control is especially important during exercise when lactic acid is accumulating. Lactic acid releases hydrogen ions, which can reduce the muscle's ability to produce ATP and can hinder the contractile process. An increase in pulmonary ventilation lowers hydrogen ion concentration through the formation of HCO_3, creating a more basic environment. A decrease in pulmonary ventilation raises hydrogen ion concentration, creating a more acidic environment. Therefore, it is important to have optimal pulmonary function during exercise.

ENERGY SYSTEMS

The importance of a balanced diet and good nutrition are well-known facts. The nutrients from food provide the necessary energy for normal bodily function. The importance of good nutrition increases as the demands of exercise increase. Fuel for exercise can come from carbohydrates, fats, or proteins. Carbohydrates (CHO) provide an immediate source of energy. One gram of CHO is equal to four kcal of energy. Carbohydrates can exist in three different forms: monosaccharides, disaccharides, or polysaccharides. Monosaccharides are simple sugars and are found as glucose, which is blood sugar; fructose, which is fruit and honey sugar; or galactose, which is milk sugar. Disaccharides consist of two monosaccharides and can take the form of sucrose (glucose and fructose), maltose (two glucose molecules), or lactose (galactose and glucose). Polysaccharides are considered complex CHO and consist of three or more monosaccharides. They are present in plants such as cellulose and starch, and in animals. Polysaccharides that are stored in animals are termed glycogen. Glycogen can be stored in muscles or in the liver. Fats are used as a prolonged energy source. One gram of fat is equal to nine kcal of energy. Simple fats, or triglycerides, are our primary fat energy source. Compound fats (phospholipids) and derived fats (cholesterol) are not used for energy. Proteins are made up of amino acids. There are at least 20 different amino acids utilized in the body. One gram of protein is equal to 4 kcal of energy. Proteins can contribute to fuel for exercise in two different ways. The amino acid alanine can be converted to glucose in the liver. Also, the amino acids isoleucine, alanine, leucine, and valine can be converted to metabolic intermediates for bioenergetic pathways in the muscle cells.

High energy phosphates serve as another immediate source of energy for the body. Adenosine triphoshate (ATP) forms a high energy bond when adenosine diphosphate (ADP) is coupled with an inorganic phosphate. When the enzyme ATPase breaks this bond, energy is released and used for work. Phosphocreatine (PC) is another high energy phosphate that is used for ATP production. When PC is coupled with ADP, it forms ATP and creatine.

The use of fuel for energy is controlled via anaerobic and aerobic metabolism. Anaerobic metabolism is the most rapid means of producing ATP, and is used without oxygen. The ATP-PC system provides energy at the onset of exercise and during short-term high-intensity exercise (< 5 seconds). This type of energy metabolism is important in high intensity exercises such as sprinting, high jump, weight lifting, and football. Glycolysis, which is the breakdown of glucose or glycogen, provides energy during the initial stages of exercise. It is utilized during moderate to high intensity exercise such as the 400-meter run.

Aerobic metabolism (also known as oxidative phosphorylation) occurs inside the mitochondria. It is used during prolonged exercise and requires oxygen. Aerobic metabolism involves the integration of two metabolic pathways, the Kreb's cycle and the electron transport system. The Kreb's cycle entails removal of hydrogen from CHO, fats, or proteins and provides energy that can be used in the electron transport chain to combine ADP and inorganic phosphate to form ATP. The electron transport system forms ATP, providing an energy source for long-term exercise. At the end of the electron transport chain, oxygen accepts electrons to combine with hydrogen and form H_2O.

The integration of circulatory and respiratory function prime the body for the use of food for energy. While only basic concepts were discussed here, the complex integration of all of these systems allow for optimal endurance training and performance. Without a basic understanding of these concepts, application to practical use is difficult. It is important to keep these basic principles in mind and refer to this chapter or other sources when applying endurance training techniques.

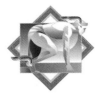

Chapter Nine

Techniques of Endurance Training

Similar to the techniques of strength training, it is important to include an appropriate warm-up and cool-down before and after endurance activities. The warm-up allows the body to ready itself for activity, and the cool-down encourages blood to flow through the body, ridding it of any exercise waste byproducts. Different endurance training techniques will be discussed in this chapter with an emphasis on training examples for each technique.

WARM-UP

We recommend beginning with a brief period of aerobic activity in order to increase heart rate, respiration rate, blood flow, muscle temperature, and joint viscosity. This allows for more effective stretching exercises and prepares the body for the upcoming training session. Examples of aerobic activity for the warm-up include brisk walking, slow jogging, cycle ergometer, or some form of calisthenics such as rope jumping, jumping jacks, or light aerobic dance. Following 5 to 7 minutes of light aerobic activity, it is important to stretch the muscles involved in the endurance exercise activity. Stretching exercises aid in preparing muscles, joints, and ligaments for the added stress of the training session. Be sure to include both upper and lower body stretches, even if the endurance activity is focused on the lower body. For example, although running seems like primarily a lower body event, the upper body is still active and involved in balance support and forward propulsion. Specific techniques of flexibility training are discussed in Chapter Fifteen.

LOW-IMPACT ACTIVITIES

Low-impact endurance activities are especially recommended for beginners, older individuals, overweight individuals, and persons susceptible to orthopedic injury. Low-impact activities generally include a type of continuous endurance training that involves minimal stress to the joints and structures of the body. They are usually lower intensity exercises performed for

a longer duration and are also known as long, slow-distance exercises (LSD). Some examples include:
1. Walking
2. Cycling
3. Swimming
4. Rowing
5. Stair climbing
6. Low-impact aerobic dance
7. Low-impact step aerobics
8. Cross-country skiing.

HIGH-IMPACT ACTIVITIES

High-impact activities involve some form of running or jumping activity. When prescribing high-impact, high intensity, high frequency, and/or prolonged duration exercises, be aware that injury rates increase exponentially. If you are prescribing high-impact endurance exercises, be sure to moderate frequency and duration. These activities may be continuous or intermittent in nature and should include short to moderate duration. Examples of high-impact activities include:
1. Jogging/running
2. Basketball
3. Volleyball
4. Jumping/hopping activities
5. Rope skipping
6. High-impact aerobic dance
7. High-impact step aerobics
8. Racquet sports.

LIFETIME SPORTS

Lifetime sports involve recreational activities that require varying levels of fitness and are often centered on group participation. These types of activities usually allow for participation at all age levels and encourage lifetime commitment to physical activity. Examples of lifetime sports include:
1. Cycling
2. Swimming
3. Dancing
4. Hiking
5. Canoeing/kayaking
6. Golf
7. Bowling.

OVER DISTANCE TRAINING

The objective of over distance training is to improve the body's ability for maximum oxygen consumption (V_{O2MAX}) and increase respiratory capacity for long duration endurance activities. It encourages the performance of an endurance activity at higher levels for long periods of time. Over distance training will also maximize the use of energy sources, in particular fat metabolism, for the support of exercise over long periods of time. Athletes who partake in over distance training regimes are marathon runners, triathletes, swimmers, cyclists, and, other ultra-distance extreme sports such as extreme hiking, climbing, and skiing. You should keep in mind, however, that over distance training does not result in sport specificity training or race pace techniques. We recommend that over distance training be incorporated with sport-specific activity in which the athlete trains the metabolic systems that support the activity and practices proper pacing techniques pertinent to the event or competition.

INTERVAL TRAINING

Interval training involves repeated bouts of exercise with brief recovery periods in between. It is an effective means of obtaining exercise overload in a short period of time. High-intensity intervals are more effective in improving aerobic power and V_{O2MAX} than low-intensity intervals. Another advantage of high-intensity interval training is that the athlete can perform more total exercise at a higher intensity than high-intensity continuous exercise. It has also been found that high-intensity interval training increases the athlete's ability to adapt to, and recover from, lactic acid accumulation. When you incorporate interval training into an endurance-training regime, the following variables must be considered. In order to improve aerobic power, the length of the work interval should be greater than 60 seconds. For sports requiring anaerobic power, this work interval may be less than 60 seconds. The rest interval should incorporate light activity, such as walking, and is often expressed as a ratio of work interval duration. It is recommended that the rest interval be at least as long as the work interval, with preferred work:rest ratios of 1:3 or 1:2. We recommend that the intensity of the work interval be 85% to 100% of maximum heart rate (MHR). During the rest interval, it is recommended that the heart rate drop to approximately 120 beats per minute. You should also consider the number of work repetitions or work intervals and the number of interval sets. For example, the athletic trainer or coach could prescribe a 200-meter run work interval at 100% intensity. He/she would then need to determine the number of repetitions such as 6 x 200-meter runs. This would equal one set. The athletic trainer may then prescribe a second set of intervals that includes a 100-meter run work interval for 10 repetitions. Another example of interval training, known as a ladder, involves using progressive durations of work for a specified number of repetitions. For example, the athletic trainer may prescribe 6 x 100-meter sprints followed by 4 x 200-meter sprints, then 2 x 400-meter sprints. This represents going up the ladder; you may also prescribe going up and down the ladder.

When prescribing interval training, one should always keep in mind the purpose of the training session and the fitness level of the athlete. For example, preseason interval training will vary as the athlete becomes more fit and progresses toward peak performance. We recommend preseason yardages for interval workouts that are between 1800 (light) to 3000 (heavy) total yards. The lighter yardage should be incorporated into the training program for at least 2 weeks before progressing to the heavier yardage. Three thousand total yards is very intense and should only be attempted by experienced athletes. Longer distance intervals are integrated early (ie, 800 yards and 400 yards), then as the athlete progresses toward the peak period (one to 2 weeks prior to the competition event or season) the interval periods are decreased. During the final two weeks, interval distances should not be above 300 yards. If interval training is incorporated two to three times a week, then the athletic trainer should incorporate light then heavy, or heavy, light, then moderate. The following example illustrates the varying yardage incorporated into an interval training program at varying points in the training regime.

EARLY PRESEASON

Heavy:	2 x 800 yards, 1 x 400 yards, 1 x 200 yards
Moderate:	3 x 400 yards, 2 x 300 yards
Light:	3 x 300 yards, 2 x 200 yards, 1 x 400 yards

MID PRESEASON

Heavy:	1 x 800 yards, 1 x 600 yards, 1 x 400 yards, 4 to 6 x 200 yards
Moderate:	2 x 400 yards, 3 x 300 yards, 2 to 4 x 200 yards
Light:	1 mile, 2 x 300 yards

PEAK PRESEASON

Heavy:	2 x 300 yards, 2 x 200 yards, 6 to 8 x 100 yards
Moderate:	4 to 6 x 200 yards
Light:	1 x 300 yards, 2 x 100 yards, 6 x 40 yards

COOL-DOWN

Following activity a cool-down is recommended. This will keep blood from pooling and encourages return of blood flow to the heart. This prevents a lack of blood flow to the brain, which can cause dizziness. An active cool-down also reduces the risk of cardiac arrhythmias, ischemia, and hypotension due to the high levels of circulating post-exercise plasma catecholamines. An active cool-down may also aid in preventing post-exercise muscle soreness by circulating metabolic waste products. The cool down period should last 5 to 10 minutes and include easy aerobic activity and light stretching exercises.

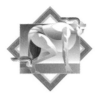

Chapter Ten

Endurance Training Exercise Prescription

The ability to sustain endurance activities is dependent upon the ability of the cardiorespiratory system to deliver, extract, and utilize oxygen. These functions are based upon the principles discussed in Chapter Eight. When prescribing endurance exercises, the athletic trainer should be familiar with some basic preliminary guidelines, which can then be applied to the four general principles of endurance training: intensity, duration, frequency, and rate of progression.

PRELIMINARY SUGGESTIONS

It is important to always begin by obtaining a medical history. Physician clearance may be needed if the athlete presents any suspicious or unusual findings. Most athletic programs incorporate a pre-participation physical examination program that provides this information along with physician clearance for all athletes. The athletic trainer should also determine physical fitness history and conduct baseline physical fitness testing to determine an athlete's present status of physical fitness. This might incorporate strength and endurance activities, along with flexibility measures and body composition measurements to determine percent body fat and fat-free body weight. Measurement of body composition can be accomplished in a variety of ways, with the most common methods including skin fold measurements and anthropometric methods that incorporate height, weight, and circumference measurements. Baseline endurance fitness testing usually involves submaximal exercise testing and heart rate monitoring. By recording an athlete's heart rate response to varying levels of submaximal exercise, the maximum level of oxygen uptake (VO2MAX) can be estimated. VO2MAX is the universal criterion for estimating cardiorespiratory fitness. Submaximal exercise tests might include the bicycle ergometer, treadmill, step test, 1-mile walk test, or Cooper's 12-minute run.

Once the trainer has determined that the athlete is healthy and has established baseline physical fitness parameters, it is important to determine the athlete's needs, interests, and objectives. Specifically, consider whether these objectives are centered on preseason versus in-season needs. Examples of pre-season versus in-season interval training workouts are presented in Chapter Nine.

Once the athlete's specific objectives have been established, set realistic short-and long-term goals. The athletic trainer may need to educate the athlete in principles of exercise technique and methods of monitoring exercise intensity and progression. Be careful not to assume the athlete has prior knowledge of exercise techniques. Just because an athlete has run before does not mean he/she runs properly. It is especially important to provide leadership and direction in the early stages of exercise. Keep in mind that the overload principle applies to endurance training, as well as strength training. Overload may be applied to training intensity, frequency, or duration.

Always remember to encourage the athletes and educate them that "more is not always better." Also, strive to dispel the myth about "no pain, no gain." Finally, it is important that you include follow-up and reevaluations of fitness status in order to modify exercise prescriptions accordingly.

INTENSITY

As mentioned earlier, maximal oxygen uptake (V_{O2MAX}) is a measure of maximal cardiorespiratory capacity and is determined via maximal and submaximal exercise testing. Direct measurement of V_{O2MAX} is obtained through the collection of expired gases and is often not feasible for the practitioner in a clinical or traditional athletic training setting. Estimating V_{O2MAX} using the heart rate response has been validated and is commonly used to prescribe endurance exercise intensity. It is well known that a linear relationship exists between heart rate (HR) and V_{O2MAX}. Endurance exercise intensity can be expressed in a variety of ways. In terms of V_{O2MAX}, the recommended intensity of endurance exercise is between 50% to 85% of V_{O2MAX}. Figure 10-1 illustrates a comparison of V_{O2MAX} values in young and middle-aged men of various fitness levels. Values for women are not presented, but they average 10% to 20% lower than men. Other methods of expressing endurance exercise intensity are discussed below.

Maximum heart rate (MHR), expressed as the number of beats per minute, is the most common method of prescribing endurance exercise intensity. MHR can be obtained directly by performing a maximum graded exercise test and monitoring the heart rate response. Again, this method of direct observation is often not feasible; therefore, a formula for predicting MHR has been established. MHR is equal to 220 minus the athlete's age (+/- 12 bpm). Endurance exercise intensity is then prescribed at 60% to 90% of MHR. For example, if you are working with a 20-year-old athlete, his/her approximate MHR = 220 – 20 or 200 bpm. Then, depending on the athlete's training goals, a percentage of his/her MHR is assigned. For example, if the athlete wanted to train at 80% of his/her MHR, he/she should work at an intensity level that elicits a heart rate of 160 bpm. Another similar method of prescribing exercise intensity is using the heart rate reserve (HRR). The HRR is equal to MHR minus the resting heart rate. Endurance exercise intensity using this method is prescribed at 50% to 85% of HRR. The heart rate can be measured at the carotid pulse by counting the number of beats in 15 seconds multiplied by 4, or by counting the number of beats in 10 seconds multiplied by 6. Referring to the 20-year-old athlete who is striving to work at an intensity level of 160

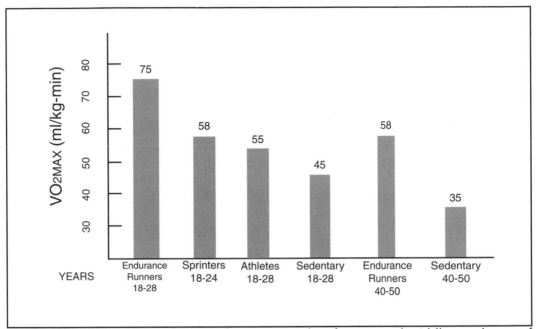

Figure 10-1. Comparison of maximal oxygen uptake of young and middle-aged men of various fitness levels. Values for women average 10% to 20% lower. (Reprinted from: Pollock ML, Wilmore JH, Fox SM. *Health and Fitness Through Physical Activity*. New York: John Wiley & Sons; 1978.)

bpm, he/she should be eliciting a 40 beat count (160/4) in 15 seconds or a 27 beat count (160/6) in 10 seconds.

Ratings of perceived exertion (RPE) are used to approximate heart rate values from rest to maximum levels of exertion, and to provide a subjective means for monitoring endurance exercise intensity. Table 10-1 identifies the various ratings of perceived exertion. The trainer would instruct the athlete to describe how the exercise is feeling at each level of exercise intensity. As noted, each feeling identified corresponds to a number on the RPE scale. This number has been shown to correlate with a corresponding HR at the same exercise intensity level. This method of prescribing exercise intensity is a valuable and reliable means of monitoring an individual's exercise tolerance.

MET or metabolic equivalent levels above resting VO_2 is another method of prescribing endurance exercise intensity. The predetermined energy costs of various physical activities are assigned in METS. One MET is equal to resting VO_2 (3.5 ml/kg/min). The recommended intensity of endurance exercise expressed in METS is equal to 50% to 85% of max METS. Low-intensity endurance exercises are categorized as less than 3.5 METS. Moderate-intensity endurance exercises are between 4 and 7 METS. Moderate to high-intensity endurance exercises are between 7 and 12 METS, while high-intensity endurance exercises are anything above 12 METS. Be advised that these ranges may vary based on individual fitness levels, age, gender, and disease.

Table 10-1

CLASSIFICATION OF INTENSITY OF EXERCISE BASED ON 30 TO 60 MINUTES OF ENDURANCE TRAINING

HRmax*	VO2 max Or HRmax Reserve*	Rating of Perceived Exertion*	Classification of Intensity
<35%	<30%	< 10	Very light
35-59%	30-49%	10-11	Light
60-79%	50-74%	12-13	Moderate
80-89%	75-84%	14-16	Heavy
>90%	>85%	>16	Very heavy

*Calculation of heart rate (HRmax), HRmax reserve, and rating of perceived exertion.

Reprinted from: Pollock ML, Wilmore JH. *Exercise in Health and Disease*. 2nd ed. Philadelphia, PA: WB Saunders Company; 1990.

Whichever method of prescribing exercise intensity is used, it is important to keep in mind the following factors:

1. Individual's level of fitness
2. Medications that influence HR
3. Risk of cardiovascular disease
4. Risk of orthopedic injury
5. Individual preferences
6. Program objectives

DURATION

The duration of endurance exercise depends on the individual athlete's level of fitness, training goals and objectives, and sport-specific requirements. High-intensity exercises performed for shorter durations are useful for high-intensity sports. We recommend that high-intensity exercises be performed intermittently for up to 5 to 10 minutes. Low-intensity exercises are performed for longer durations and may last 20 to 60 minutes. Sedentary individuals or athletes who have not participated in any activity for more than 6 months may start at durations of 5 to 10 minutes.

FREQUENCY

The frequency of exercise is dependent on both intensity and duration, in addition to the athlete's goals and lifestyle demands. Exercise improvements can occur with as few as two sessions per week, with the benefits leveling off after three to five sessions per week. Individuals who are interested in exercise for weight control should exercise five sessions per week. It is important to incorporate rest for recovery after exercise. This is especially important after intense exercise or long duration exercises, such as competitions or long-distance events. It is also very important to avoid overtraining. As mentioned, the benefits of training level off after three to five sessions. Training frequencies of more than five sessions per week are not only unproductive, but will most likely lead to injury.

RATE OF PROGRESSION

The rate of progression for endurance training depends on the athlete's health status, age, fitness level, and individual preferences and goals. When considering the rate of progression, there are typically three distinct stages that appear as follows:

1. Initial conditioning stage (lasts 4 to 6 weeks)
    a.   Intensity—50% to 70% of MHR
    b.   Duration—12 to 15 minutes up to 20 minutes
    c.   Frequency—3 times per week on alternating days
2. Improvement stage (lasts 4 to 5 months)
    a.   Intensity—60% to 90% of MHR
    b.   Duration—20 to 30 minutes
    c.   Frequency—depends on individual goals
3. Maintenance stage (begins after 6 months of training)
    a.   Reassess goals
    b.   Maintain intensity, duration, and frequency
    c.   Incorporate variety; participate in enjoyable activities

Remember to continually reevaluate the athlete's goals and document fitness gains. Exercise prescription is an evolutionary process and should be modified according to the needs of each athlete. The needs of athletes with special considerations are outlined in Chapters Seven and Twelve.

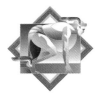

Chapter Eleven

Techniques of Speed Training

Developing speed can be accomplished in many ways. The training technique that is chosen should be individualized for the athlete and the sport in which he/she is participating. Some sports rely completely on how fast the athlete is able to move for a given distance or how fast he/she is able to change direction while maintaining speed, whereas others require speed to propel either themselves or an object. Regardless of the sport, however, every athlete must be taught the proper form and technique of running. Sprinting may not be the main focus of the sport, but applying it in training sessions will carry over onto the practice field.

FORM RUNNING

Like strength training, an adequate base must be obtained prior to engaging in sprint training sessions. A good aerobic foundation will enable the athlete to complete the high-volume, low-intensity workouts without complications.

Ensure the training surface is free of debris and adequate for running. Next inspect the footwear to see that there is good support and it is free of abnormal wear patterns. If this is apparent, the athlete may need advice from the Certified Athletic Trainer for options in maintaining correct foot mechanics. While the athlete is performing an adequate warm-up and stretch routine, measure distances of 20 and 60 yards. Form running drills 1 through 11 will utilize the 20-yard distance; 12 through 14 will use the distance of 60 yards. The drill will continue up to the yard mark; the athlete will then walk back to the original starting point. Perform one to three repetitions of each of the following drills.

Arm swing: Eyes and shoulders remain forward throughout drill. The hands are held slightly open. Forward arm is held at 90 degrees of elbow flexion as the arms rhythmically swing forward. The angle increases slightly as the arm swings backward down toward the hip.

March with high knees: As the arms swing, the leg that is opposite the forward arm simultaneously is flexing to initiate the drive into the ground. During this swing phase, the arm is forward while the hip and knee are flexed to 90 degrees. As the arms switch and are brought down toward the hip during the stance phase, the hip and knee are extended and the foot is pushed into the ground.

Quick skip: Using the above technique (with arm swing), incorporate leaving the ground slightly. Feet should land together simultaneously, not as in a regular skip in which there is a one foot landing. The skip is from one leg, but both feet are brought together during the stance phase (as in jumping over an obstacle, landing with both feet, but little distance and height is covered). This forces the drive (flexing) leg to return to the starting point quickly.

High knee lifts: Flex and drive alternating knees, landing on one foot at a time.

Skip with alternating high knee: An extra hop is introduced in the above skip method (still using arms). The skip is from one leg. While the knee flexes past 90 degrees, the first hop occurs. As the feet land, they hop simultaneously and are staggered slightly.

Skip with high knee: The same leg is repeatedly used to 10 yards, then switch to other leg.

Skip with alternating extended leg: Rather than drive a flexed knee up, flex the hip keeping the knee extended. Flex the knee slightly during landing to absorb shock.

Skip with extended leg: The same leg is repeatedly used to 10 yards, then switch to other leg.

Skip with alternating knee extension: Using the skip with high knee (and arm swing) technique, extend the knee and kick forward (during first hop) before landing (second hop, feet staggered) simultaneously.

Skip with knee extension: The same leg is repeatedly used to 10 yards, then switch to other leg.

Quick flexes: Quads remain perpendicular to the ground, while knees flex quickly and maximally. Arm swing is still emphasized in this drill. Heels should touch the gluteus maximus.

Quick flexes to jog/stride: Quick flex technique to 10 yards, jog from 10 to 40 yards, stride (increase stride length) to 60 yards.

Jog/stride: Jog (maintaining form) to 20 yards, stride from 20 to 60 yards.

Jog/stride/sprint: Jog to 10 yards, stride from 10 to 40 yards, sprint to 60 yards.

STRIDE FREQUENCY AND LENGTH

The product of stride length and frequency determines speed. Mastering the form techniques and increasing whole-body flexibility will directly determine the length of stride. Whole-body flexibility is important because an inflexible upper extremity will hinder adequate arm swing and misuse energy stores. Strength and plyometric training (discussed in Chapter Six) will produce greater frequency due to the muscle's ability to generate great force more rapidly. Always perform speed training sessions at the beginning of the conditioning workout and remember to keep training goals consistent in speed versus endurance days.

A couple of suggestions to increase stride length after adequate form has been achieved are:

1. Running downhill at approximately 3 to 7 degree slope.
2. Being towed or pulled by a partner during stride to sprint drills.

Running downhill should be performed in a safe area free of obstacles and should not cover a distance more than 60 to 80 yards. Focus on form and allow full recovery between repetitions. Discontinue the drill if fatigue begins to change the technique. Perform five to 10 repetitions. To tow or pull, fasten tubing or a harness to the athlete's chest. Tension is created in the apparatus and as the athlete begins to stride, he/she is pulled so the lean and stride length are increased. The athlete will only be able to perform approximately eight to 12 strides before tension is decreased. As in the downhill running, perform five to 10 repetitions, focus on form, allow for recovery, and discontinue as the technique begins to alter.

The use of resistance may also be implemented to increase stride and frequency. However, specificity is the key to carry over. Do not overload the athlete so much that he/she exhibits emphasis on strength. Speed training will incorporate the strength from the weight room and power from the plyometrics (see Chapter Six). Equipment such as wrist, ankle, or vest weights should be kept light and should not give the athlete a heavy feeling. A cable harness, parachute, rubber tubing, or weighted sled can be fastened to the back of the athlete to provide slight resistance. Incorporating uphill running is an effective and inexpensive resistance technique to use for all levels, especially for young and beginning participants.

As in strength training in the weight room, individualism, adequate supervision, and instruction are the ingredients for an efficient and effective speed training session. Continue to monitor and evaluate the progress of each athlete to increase productivity and decrease the incidence of injury.

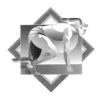

Chapter Twelve

Special Populations

DIABETIC ATHLETE

Diabetes mellitus is a chronic metabolic disease in which the mechanisms for insulin production or insulin usage are abnormal and ultimately lead to elevated blood glucose levels. Because insulin is an important hormone involved in the regulation of glucose, fat, and protein metabolism, it is imperative that you understand the management issues related to the treatment and control of this disease. More common in athletics is insulin-dependent diabetes; therefore, the focus of this section will be on the management of balancing insulin injections with food intake, and performance of rigorous blood glucose monitoring in the insulin-dependent diabetic.

There are primarily two types of diabetes, type 1 and type 2. Type 1 diabetes is also known as insulin-dependent diabetes mellitus and generally appears in persons younger than 30 years of age. Because this disease usually afflicts persons who are relatively young (ie, infants, adolescents, and young adults), it is often referred to as juvenile-onset diabetes. Type 1 diabetes is the most common type for persons who participate in athletics or sport; however, this type of diabetes represents only 5% to 10% of the diabetic population. Type 1 diabetics lack the ability to secrete insulin from the pancreas and are required to use insulin injections or pumps in order to control blood glucose levels. Resting blood glucose levels for the average individual range from 80 to 115 mg/dl, whereas the diabetic individual may have high, low, or normal levels. Type 2 diabetes is also known as noninsulin-dependent diabetes mellitus and represents approximately 90% to 95% of all diabetics. It is usually found in adults over the age of 30; however, in some cases it may occur in a younger population as well. Type 2 diabetes is generally related to one of the following risk factors: obesity, older age, family history of diabetes, physical inactivity, and ethnic origin, specifically Native American, African American, Hispanic American, and Asian and Pacific Island American. The pathophysiology of type 2 diabetes is multifaceted, and some aspects of it are still not understood. Nevertheless, the consequences of this disease are focused toward decreased insulin action and require that these individuals undergo various forms of treatment to control their blood glucose, such as dietary intervention, exercise, use of oral medication, and/or insulin injections. Regardless of the type of diabetes, all diabetics are at risk for serious health problems and premature death. Therefore, it is essential that persons with diabetes be familiar with the management of their disease, perform regular self blood glucose monitoring (SBGM) tests, and strive to maintain a healthy lifestyle. An athletic trainer should also become familiar with blood glucose monitoring and keep a log of blood glucose responses in diabetic athletes. This will enable the athletic trainer to understand how each athlete responds to his/her individual exercise and/or training program.

Exercise is one part of maintaining a healthy lifestyle and can enhance the efficiency of biochemical and metabolic processes that help to maintain blood glucose levels in diabetic individuals. It is important for athletic trainers to ensure that the diabetic athlete has controlled blood glucose levels prior to exercise and has taken an adequate amount of insulin. Through exercise, the controlled diabetic can influence the release of liver glucose, enhance glucose uptake by the muscles, and decrease blood glucose levels. This may decrease the medication requirement, lead to a reduction in body fat, provide valuable cardiovascular benefits, reduce stress, and aid in the prevention of type 2 diabetes.

When recommending exercise for the diabetic athlete, you should individualize the program according to presence and severity of the disease and associated complications, medication schedule, and goals of the athlete. As with any athlete, pre-participation screening is recommended for the diabetic athlete. In regard to the diabetic athlete, it is important to screen for microvascular (eg, kidney function or eye damage), macrovascular (eg, coronary artery disease [CAD]), peripheral vascular disease, and cerebrovascular disease), and neurological complications. If CAD is present or suspected, an exercise electrocardiogram is recommended prior to the start of any physical activity. Even with pre-participation approval from a physician, diabetics should have regular medical check-ups that assess metabolic control and current health status related to any diabetic complication.

An important component of exercise programming is balancing exercise activities with dietary and medication schedules. If the diabetic begins exercise with markedly decreased levels of insulin, he/she will have an increased release of liver glucose and decreased glucose uptake by the muscle, resulting in increased blood glucose levels or hyperglycemia. Hyperglycemia causes excessive ketones to be broken down via fatty acid metabolism, which ultimately contributes to diabetic ketoacidosis (DKA). If metabolic control is ignored for several consecutive days, DKA causes diabetics to go into a coma and is potentially life threatening. If the diabetic begins exercise with too much insulin, he/she will have a marked increase in glucose uptake by the muscle and decreased glucose release from liver, resulting in decreased blood glucose levels. This can lead to a dangerous hypoglycemic response. Therefore, diabetics should balance exercise by increasing carbohydrate intake and decreasing injected insulin prior to exercise. The following recommendations are provided for safely participating in exercise and avoiding excessive lows and highs in blood glucose. The athlete should assess blood glucose levels before and after each exercise session. This is especially important for the "newly diagnosed" type 1 diabetic. Every individual's glucose response to exercise is different and it is always better to err on the side of knowing too much, rather than too little. Proper management depends upon balancing exercise with diet, insulin (for those diabetics requiring insulin), and SBGM.

If the athlete is involved in leisure activity and his/her blood glucose level is less than 100 mg $\times$ dl-1, then there is no need to increase carbohydrate intake prior to exercise.

If the athlete is involved in moderate activity and his/her blood glucose level is 100 to 180 mg × dl-1, then 10 to 15 gm of carbohydrates should be eaten prior to exercise. If blood glucose levels are 180 to 300 mg × dl-1, there is no need to increase carbohydrate intake. If the blood glucose level is greater than 300 mg×dl-1, then exercise is not recommended. If the athlete is going to engage in intense activity for 1 to 2 hours and has an acceptable blood glucose level, then 25 to 50 gm of carbohydrates should be eaten prior to exercise.

Other recommendations include:

- Avoiding insulin injections in exercising muscles prior to exercise
- Carbohydrate consumption post exercise to replenish muscle glycogen stores and avoid post exercise hypoglycemia
- Increase fluid intake before, during, and after exercise
- Carry a readily available source of carbohydrates
- Wear medical tags identifying diabetic condition
- Avoid exercising alone
- Avoid exercising when ill or infection is present
- Avoid exercising in extreme temperatures
- Wear proper footwear
- Inspect feet daily and after exercise
- Regular medical check-ups to assess health status and presence of common diabetic complications.

The principles of training frequency, duration, and rate of progression outlined in Chapter Ten are similar for the diabetic individual. However, it is recommended that the intensity of endurance exercise be moderated in the type 2 diabetic individual. Intensity ranges may be modified to 50% to 74% of maximal aerobic capacity for the type 2 diabetic. Type 1 diabetics are more apt to be able to exercise at higher intensities without incidence. Also recommended for the elite athlete is to keep a careful training log that includes exercise activity (type, duration, and intensity of exercise) along with food ingestion, medication dosages, SBGM values, and site of insulin injections. This will aid in coordinating an intensive training schedule and allow for adjustments in diet, exercise activity, and medication dosages as needed.

EXERCISE-INDUCED ASTHMA

Asthma is a respiratory disorder brought on by an allergen, irritant, or exercise that affects breathing capacity. The allergen, irritant, or exercise triggers the smooth muscle in the bronchioles to constrict, which results in increased resistance in the bronchiole tubes and makes breathing difficult. In addition, secretions of mucous from cells in the bronchiole walls further compromises air exchange in the lungs. Exercise-induced asthma (EIA) is bronchospasms in the bronchioles brought on specifically by exercise. EIA is more commonly seen in individuals diagnosed with asthma. The signs and symptoms of asthma include coughing, wheezing, increased mucous production, chest tightness, shortness of breath, and fatigue.

EIA can be caused by:
1. Cold, dry air
2. Hypocapnia (low partial pressure CO_2)
3. Respiratory alkalosis
4. Strenuous exercise
5. Long duration exercise
6. Improper use of asthma medication

Typically, the asthma attack occurs within 6 to 12 minutes of exercise or may appear 5 to 10 minutes after cessation of the exercise activity. Therefore, it is important for individuals with EIA to include a proper warm-up and cool-down period with their exercise program.

When treating EIA, one should not underestimate the benefits that exercise can offer an individual with asthma. However, it is important to control the disorder and follow some simple recommended guidelines. The recommended pharmacological management of EIA includes the use of b2 agonist inhalers, which serve as a short-acting treatment, and/or the use of prescribed prophylactic medications such as theophylline or cromolyn sodium. The recommended dosages for exercise are as follows:

1. Athletes with normal airway function
   a. Administer b2 agonist or cromolyn sodium 10 minutes prior to exercise or competition
   b. Ingest 5 mg × kg-1 of rapid release theophylline 1 hour prior to exercise
2. Athletes with abnormal airway function
   a. Administer b2 agonist or cromolyn sodium 10 minutes prior to exercise or competition
   b. Ingest 12 to 20 mg × kg-1×d-1 of sustained release theophylline

Other important guidelines include:
1. Incorporate gradual exercise progression
2. Exercise in a warm, humid environment (eg, swimming)
3. If exercising in cold, dry environment wear scarf or face mask to moisten air
4. Keep inhaler with b2 agonist readily available
5. Avoid other asthma triggers during exercise
6. Avoid exercising alone
7. Utilize diaphragmatic breathing
8. Incorporate interval training for high-intensity exercises
9. Be aware of the early signs of an asthma attack, then modify or discontinue the exercise activity as necessary
10. If the athlete is competing, be aware of medications that might appear on a banned substance list with the competition organization.

WOMEN

While women are becoming more and more active physically and participating in competitive sports, there is still much needed research on the benefits of physical activity in women. Women respond equally as well to endurance training as men, except during the luteal phase of the menstrual cycle when exercise thermoregulation is impaired. During the luteal phase of menstruation, women tend to sweat less and have higher heart rates and core body temperatures than men when involved in light to moderate exercise. The luteal phase of menstruation occurs right after ovulation; women who are exercising in extreme temperatures should be aware of their cycle and modify activity as needed. The primary concern for a female athlete is a phenomenon known as the "female athlete triad." The female athlete triad identifies three different health problems that are surprisingly interrelated in this population. These health problems include: amenorrhea, eating disorders, and bone mineral loss.

Intense endurance training, specifically distance running, affects the length of the menstrual cycle, and may lead to amenorrhea, which is a lack of menstruation (< four menses/year). Amenorrhea is most often associated with high training mileage and low body fat percentages. In addition to long-distance runners, ballet dancers and gymnasts appear to be susceptible, most likely due to the emphasis on low body fat percentages. High training mileage alters blood hormone concentrations and affects hypothalamus feedback and the release of reproductive hormones. Additionally, training that brings on psychological stress is thought to disrupt the menstrual cycle by increasing catecholamine and/or endogenous opiate levels, which play a role in regulating reproductive systems. Amenorrheic women have been shown to have a delayed metabolism response when exposed to colder temperatures. The reason for this is uncertain and cannot be explained by differences in body fat. Ultimately, the presence of amenorrhea leads to low levels of estradiol. Over time, this will lead to a decrease in bone mineral content and premature osteoporosis. Dysmenorrhea, or painful menstruation, is also thought to be higher in athletic populations than nonathletic populations. This may be due to the release of prostaglandins with exercise; these cause smooth muscle in the uterus to contract, resulting in ischemia and pain. If severe, the pain can be treated with antiprostaglandin drugs.

Certain female sports place a heavy emphasis on body weight and percent fat. Specifically, ballet dancing, gymnastics, ice skating, swimming, diving, and body building are sports in which there is a high occurrence of eating disorders. It is important for athletic trainers and coaches to be aware of the signs and symptoms of anorexia nervosa and bulimia nervosa, two types of eating disorders. Bulimia is characterized by an abnormal and constant craving for food that results in a food binging/purging cycle. Excessive purging will result in a loss of electrolytes, which can lead to poor thermoregulation and physical performance. Anorexia is a form of self starvation. If left untreated, it can lead to death. Through careful observation and guidance throughout a female's athletic career, these disorders can be prevented and serious health complications can be avoided. Figures 12-1 and 12-2 identify the warning signs of anorexia nervosa and bulimia. Female athletes who have an eating disorder or even episodes of altered eating behavior are at risk for inadequate nutritional intake and, in particular, low calcium intake. This only adds to the problem of amenorrhea and the potential for bone mineral loss. If the athletic trainer suspects that an athlete has an eating disorder, care should be taken in how the athlete is approached. Someone who is trusted, with whom the athlete does not feel embarrassed, is usually the best person. The goal in approaching the athlete is to convince her to seek counseling, preferably psychological counseling, and in some cases nutritional counseling. Be careful not to allow gossip among team members and consider the use

Figure 12-1. The warning signs of anorexia nervosa. (Reprinted from: Powers SK, Howley ET. *Exercise Physiology.* 3rd ed. Dubuque, IA: Brown & Benchmark Publishers; 1997.)

Figure 12-2. The warning signs of bulimia nervosa. (Reprinted from: Powers SK, Howley ET. *Exercise Physiology.* 3rd ed. Dubuque, IA: Brown & Benchmark Publishers; 1997.)

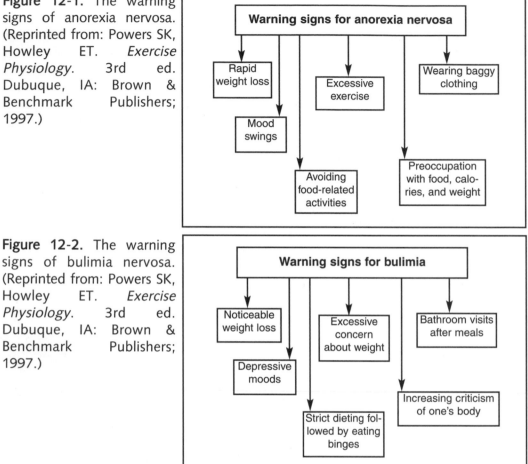

of an eating disorder inventory with the entire team. Although women are discussed here in regard to eating disorders, the athletic trainer should not disregard male sports that emphasize body weight and percent of fat, such as wrestling, distance running, crew, and gymnastics.

The combination of intense training and the pressure to maintain low body weight and body fat for certain types of sports lends itself to a dangerous result: premature osteoporosis. As mentioned, the presence of amenorrhea brought on by intense training negatively impacts the quality of bone density. Furthermore, the lack of calcium intake associated with poor eating habits and restricted caloric intake only exacerbates the potential for bone mineral loss. Over time, these factors will lead to premature osteoporosis. Females that begin training at an early age, especially prepubescents and adolescents, are at an even greater risk of premature osteoporosis if diet and training regimes are not closely monitored over time. The cumulative effects of intense training and poor eating habits over time are exacerbated when women begin training early in life. As a strength and conditioning specialist, one should be especially aware of the detrimental impacts of the "female athlete triad" and include appropriate preventative measures, as well as necessary referral methods.

Women are also subject to low levels of iron due to iron loss in sweat and during menstruation. The repetitive pounding associated with long-distance running may cause hemolysis of red blood cells, resulting in loss of hemoglobin through urine. It is also thought that athletes are not as apt to absorb dietary iron as compared to sedentary individuals. Serum ferritin may also be deficient in female athletes. It is recommended that female athletes take an iron supplement on a regular basis. Female runners are recommended to take 18 mg of supplemental iron per day, in addition to having their serum ferritin level checked each year.

SENIORS

As mentioned with strength training, there are physiological changes that occur with age. Reportedly, aerobic capacity decreases with age as measured by VO2MAX. These changes are associated with numerous physiological declines and are outlined in Table 12-1. The rate of decline is dependent upon cardiorespiratory fitness level and certain disease conditions. In fact, endurance exercise may slow the rate of decline and even reverse decreases in aerobic capacity in elderly populations. Older individuals, who have been active throughout life, respond better to cardiovascular adaptations than older individuals who have been sedentary throughout life.

Endurance exercise is said to aid in preventing osteoporosis by maintaining bone structure through the force of gravity seen with upright posture and forces of muscle contraction. In particular, physical activity that incorporates muscle contraction and weightbearing activity is thought to deliver mechanical loading to the bones that result in increased bone mineral density. Weightbearing activities (eg, walking and jogging) are better for maintaining bone mineral content than non weightbearing activities (eg, swimming and cycling). However, it is important that sedentary individuals or those with previous fractures begin with non weightbearing activities, then progress to weightbearing activities as tolerated. In particular, individuals with osteoporosis are at risk for osteoporotic fractures and should be careful when performing certain exercises. Falls in this population are dangerous in that they can lead to serious health complications and premature death. Low-intensity, low-impact exercise that encourages balance performance and training is ideal for the prevention of falls which can lead to fractures and associated complications.

It is always advised that older individuals obtain physician clearance prior to beginning any exercise program. As with any population, we recommend that older individuals incorporate a comprehensive warm-up and cool-down period that focuses on flexibility training. The greatest benefits of exercise occur when a combination of flexibility, balance, strength, and endurance exercises are performed. Generally, the primary objectives of prescribing exercise for seniors are to increase functional capacity and independence and slow the effects of aging. When prescribing exercises for the older individual, keep in mind the following parameters:
1. Intensity
    a. Better to use measured maximum heart rate (MHR) than age-predicted MHR
    b. Use percentage of HR reserve or rating of perceived exertion (RPE) for prescribing intensity (recommended 50% to 70% HR reserve or RPE)
2. Duration

Table 12-1

PHYSIOLOGICAL CHANGES ASSOCIATED WITH AGING

System	Function	Change
Cardiovascular	Resting Heart Rate	No change
	Maximal Heart Rate	Decrease
	Resting Cardiac Output	Decrease
	Maximal Cardiac Output	Decrease
	Resting Stroke Volume	Decrease
	Maximal Stroke Volume	Decrease
	Resting Blood Pressure	Increase
	Exercise Blood Pressure	Increase
	Maximal Oxygen Consumption	Decrease
Respiratory	Residual Volume	Increase
	Vital Capacity	Decrease
	Total Lung Capacity	No Change
	Respiratory Frequency	Increase
Nervous	Reaction Time	Decrease
	Nerve Conduction Time	Increase
	Sensory Deficits	Increase
Musculoskeletal	Muscular Strength	Decrease
	Muscle Mass	Decrease
	Flexibility	Decrease
	Balance	Decrease
	Bone Density	Decrease
Renal	Kidney Function	Decrease
	Acid-Base Control	Decrease
	Glucose Tolerance	Decrease
	Drug Clearance	Decrease
	Cellular Water	Decrease
Metabolic	Basal Metabolic Rate	Decrease
	Lean Body Mass	Decrease
	Body Fat	Increase

Reprinted from: American College of Sports Medicine. *ACSM's Exercise Management for Persons with Chronic Diseases and Disabilities*. Champaign, Ill: Human Kinetics; 1997.

   a. If unable to sustain 20 minutes of aerobic exercise, perform several bouts of 5 to 10 minute exercise sessions throughout the day

   b. As exercise program progresses, increase duration before intensity

3. Frequency

      a. Emphasize gradual progression and adequate rest; older individuals adapt to the stresses of exercise much slower than younger individuals

      b. Alternate between weightbearing and non weightbearing activities

4. Type of exercise

      a. Older individuals should avoid high-impact activities and overtraining; rate of injury increases exponentially

      b. Include convenient, enjoyable, and accessible activities

      c. Recommended—walking, stationary cycling, water exercises, swimming, stair climbing (machine), and chair exercises

5. Other recommendations

      a. Be aware of the individual's current medication history; some medications produce side effects that may contraindicate certain types of exercise

      b. Be aware of medical history and associated concerns such as previous injury, presence of osteoarthritis, and possible joint replacement surgeries

      c. Encourage adequate hydration

      d. Educate older persons on how to monitor their heart rate; if the individual is participating in a supervised exercise program consider also blood pressure monitoring

      e. Have an emergency plan in place and post it in view of all participants and supervising personnel

      f. Include motivational techniques to encourage consistent and committed participation; this population responds well to social activities and goal/reward programs.

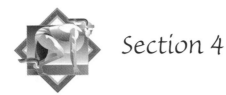

Section 4

Nutritional Aids For Sports Performance

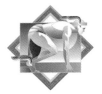 *Chapter Thirteen*

Basic Dietary Recommendations for Athletes

Mark Kern, PhD, RD

IMPORTANCE OF AN ADEQUATE DIET FOR PERFORMANCE

While there is no substitute for genetic endowment and rigorous training in the achievement of optimal athletic performance, sound nutrition is vital for maximizing athletic potential. The importance of proper dietary intake for athletes has been recognized for centuries, yet the modern field of sports nutrition is still very young and there is much to be learned about using foods and dietary supplements for achieving peak performance. Although controversies persist on how diet may provide the winning edge, few researchers or dietitians would argue against the notion that an inadequate diet, deficient in energy or essential nutrients, will impair performance.

The key to proper nutrition is the consumption of a natural, wholesome diet providing a variety of foods from each of the major food groups. Following a balanced dietary regimen is important not only for optimizing performance, but also to prevent chronic diseases, such as heart disease, stroke, cancer, and diabetes, which are related to poor eating practices. Many nutritional guidelines such as the Food Guide Pyramid and the *Dietary Guidelines for Americans* are available to the athlete, athletic trainer, and coach to assist in making wise food selections. The 1995 edition of the *Dietary Guidelines for Americans*, published jointly by the United States Department of Agriculture (USDA) and Department of Health and Human Services, provides seven sensible practices that can serve as foundations for healthy eating. These guidelines include the following.

1) Eat a variety of foods.
2) Balance the food you eat with physical activity to maintain or improve your weight.
3) Choose a diet with plenty of grain products, vegetables, and fruits.
4) Choose a diet low in fat, saturated fat, and cholesterol.
5) Choose a diet moderate in sugars.
6) Choose a diet moderate in salt and sodium.
7) If you drink alcoholic beverages, do so in moderation.

Figure 13-1. Food Guide Pyramid. (Reprinted from: US Department of Agriculture/US Department of Health and Human Services.)

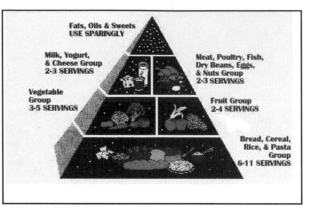

The USDA's Food Guide Pyramid provides a more specific set of recommendations for consuming an adequate diet without excess intake of energy, fat, saturated fat, cholesterol, sugars, sodium, and alcohol. The Food Guide Pyramid was developed as a practical representation of food selection for the *Dietary Guidelines for Americans.* Although more specific than the *Dietary Guidelines*, a major strength of the Pyramid is that it allows the user a high degree of freedom to make selections that fit his or her personal beliefs, tastes, financial status, and other factors affecting dietary intake. Figure 13-1 is a summary of the Pyramid's recommendations for intake.

Portion sizes used as the foundations for the range of recommended servings often vary from the typical servings used by individual athletes. For example, some athletes may consume 1 to 2 cups or more of pasta during a meal and consider it one serving from the bread, cereal, rice, and pasta group, when in fact, the Food Guide Pyramid considers this to be two to four or more servings. Clearly, an athlete using his or her own self-selected serving sizes may have difficulty using the Pyramid as a diet aid. A basic guide for what constitutes a serving from each food group is provided in Table 13-1.

Through consuming a variety of foods at the suggested serving size, eating the lowest number of servings in the range for each food group will typically result in an energy intake of approximately 1600 kcals. The upper level of each range typically results in a daily intake of approximately 2800 kcals. The number of servings needed by an individual athlete depends on his or her energy expenditure, which in turn depends on a wide variety of factors such as age, gender, weight, and activity level, as well as many other variables. Due to the increased energy expenditure of exercise training, many athletes need to consume more food than would be provided by the upper range of servings from each group. For these athletes, a proportionally higher intake from each group, focussing on the bread, vegetable, and fruit groups, is needed to ensure adequate energy and nutrient intake.

A visit to the following websites can provide further detail on using these guides for sound nutritional practices. The reader can also find an expanded list of serving size suggestions for the Food Guide Pyramid.

•*Dietary Guidelines for Americans*: www.usda.gov/cnpp/guide.htm
•*Food Guide Pyramid*: www.usda.gov/cnpp/pyramid2.htm

With respect to the relative proportions of major nutrients providing energy from the diet (fat, carbohydrate, and protein), optimal intake for performance is unclear. However, most

Table 13-1

TYPICAL SERVING SIZES FROM THE MAJOR FOOD GROUPS OF THE FOOD GUIDE PYRAMID

Food Group	Typical Serving Sizes
Bread, Cereal, Rice, and Pasta Group	1 slice bread ½ bun or English muffin 1 small roll, biscuit, or muffin ½ cup cooked cereal, rice, or pasta 1 ounce breakfast cereal
Vegetable Group	½ cup cooked vegetables ½ cup chopped raw vegetables 1 cup leafy raw vegetables ¾ cup vegetable juice
Fruit Group	1 medium fruit item (eg, apple, banana, orange) ½ cup chopped, cooked, or canned fruit or whole berries 1 melon wedge ¼ cup dried fruit ¾ cup fruit juice
Meat, Poultry, Fish, Dry Beans, Eggs, and Nuts Group	2-3 ounces cooked lean meat, poultry, or fish 1 egg = 1 ounce of meat ½ cup cooked beans = 1 ounce meat 2 tablespoons peanut butter = 1 ounce meat
Milk, Yogurt, and Cheese Group	1 cup milk 8 ounces yogurt 1½ ounces natural cheese 2 ounces processed cheese

sports nutritionists recommend consuming the majority of calories (at least 55% to 60% of kcals) from carbohydrates to help maintain stores of carbohydrates in the body, which when depleted, can lead to fatigue. Fat consumption should be limited to less than 30% of kcals to: 1) allow for a higher relative carbohydrate intake, 2) prevent chronic diseases, and 3) decrease risk of excess calorie consumption that can result in unwanted weight gain. Although protein needs are greater for athletes than nonathletes, usual recommendations based on energy intake are consistent between the two groups (12% to 15% of kcals) since energy intake is likely higher for athletes. Along with increased energy intake in athletes versus nonathletes, which usually occurs due to higher energy expenditure, grams of protein consumed automatically increases if the percent of calories obtained from protein remains constant. Results of several studies vary, but current research suggests that protein requirements of endurance athletes range between 1.0 to 1.6 g/kg and of strength athletes range between 1.2 to 1.8 g/kg.

TWO MAJOR CONSIDERATIONS FOR OPTIMAL PERFORMANCE

Much research in the field of sports nutrition has been conducted on food components that can optimize performance. Most experts on sports nutrition would agree that research has determined that two dietary factors—adequate fluid and carbohydrate intake—can enhance performance in many athletic events.

Adequate Hydration

Adequate fluid intake during training or an event is crucial to prevent the decrease in work capacity that accompanies dehydration. Studies have suggested that the loss of as little as between 1% to 2% of body weight via dehydration can hinder performance. During competition this hindrance can mean losing the event; thus consumption of adequate fluids before and during performance is critical. Dehydration during training may also lead to impaired performance by diminishing the athletes' ability to train at the highest possible level, resulting in suboptimal fitness and preparation for competition.

Fluid requirements vary with several factors including sport/event, exercise intensity, duration of exercise bout, and climate; therefore, it is impossible to provide all athletes with a single recommendation for fluid needed for competition. However, general recommendations of the American College of Sports Medicine are to consume .5 liters of fluid approximately 2 hours prior to exercise and to drink adequate fluids at regular intervals during exercise to replace fluids lost through sweat. Plain water is likely all that is needed during events lasting less than 1 hour; however, athletes often fail to adequately maintain hydration during exercise in both long and short events. In this case, a major role for the athletic trainer can be to optimize fluid intake by providing or suggesting the use of the most palatable fluids possible. Suggestions may include use of: 1) cool fluids (between 15°-22° C), 2) flavored beverages, 3) sweetened beverages, and 4) beverages that include sodium (about 0.5 g/l of fluid). Studies have shown that each of these factors can enhance fluid intake, thus decreasing the likelihood of dehydration during an event. These suggestions become progressively more important during longer events, but may also stimulate more adequate fluid consumption during short events for which plain water is usually sufficient. Most chilled commercial sports drinks on the market have these qualities and will likely enhance intake. Sports drinks that are carbonated may exhibit these characteristics as well; however, athletic trainers should use caution when recommending these beverages because some research indicates that fluid consumption may be lower due to gastric expansion caused by the carbonation.

Adequate Carbohydrate Intake

Adequate carbohydrate intake before and/or during an event, particularly 1) rigorous endurance events lasting approximately 1 hour or longer, 2) events that include intermittent bursts of high intensity activity, and 3) events performed in cold environments, can enhance performance. Research indicates that dietary carbohydrates provide an alternate fuel source that can spare the use of the body's carbohydrate stores, thus prolonging time to fatigue. Carbohydrate needs vary with athlete preference, sport, or event in which he or she is participating and timing of intake relative to competition. A basic recommendation for carbohydrate consumption prior to an event is to consume 4 to 5 g/kg about 4 hours before the start of the event. The athlete should experiment with different food sources, possibly including commercial carbohydrate supplements, to determine which food selections will work best to achieve this level of intake. Research has also shown that closer to the event, approximately 1 to 2 g/kg consumed 1 hour prior to the event may improve performance, and consumption of 50 to 60 g immediately before the event may prolong endurance. During an event it is generally recommended that an athlete consume approximately 8 ounces of a 5% to 10% carbohydrate solution every 15 minutes. This schedule is clearly not possible for all sports and events and should be adjusted for the individual athlete in a manner that is appropriate for his/her particular competition. The source of the carbohydrate is likely a secondary factor, but some research indicates that different sources of carbohydrates may have varying effects on the body's physiology and performance. Foods that promote faster entry of carbohydrates into the blood stream may prove useful during and after an event, while optimal pre-event meals may include foods that promote a slower entry. More research is needed to determine what type of carbohydrate is best for various occasions.

OTHER DIETARY CONSIDERATIONS

The scope of this text does not allow for a complete discussion of all aspects of sports nutrition; however, the previous discussion of basic recommendations and adequate fluid and carbohydrate intake covers what most experts perceive to be the most critical aspects of the athletes' dietary needs. Other considerations do exist, although they likely are of less importance to optimal performance, are applicable to fewer athletes, and/or are not as fully understood. Presented here are some concerns that athletic trainers often must address.

Pregame Meals

Many athletes ignore regular consumption of a healthy diet and instead place great importance only on the pregame or pre-event meal. Although a good pregame meal cannot replace good overall dietary habits, it can remain an important adjunct to adequate daily intake. Williams has outlined a few guidelines that should be used by athletes during the meal before competition. These recommendations include consuming a meal composed of foods that will allow the stomach to be relatively empty before the event. The meal should be high in carbohydrates and low in fiber, fat, and protein and should usually be eaten approximately 3 to 4 hours before competition. Liquid meals (eg, GatorPro, Boost, Ensure, etc) are often less likely to cause gastrointestinal disturbances (ie cramps, gas, nausea, and/or diarrhea) and may be consumed closer to the event (eg, 2 to 3 hours prior). Consuming a liquid meal may be the best choice for early morning events that begin relatively soon after waking. Personal preference based on taste, adequate energy and water content, and absence of gastrointestinal disturbances should be the major factors in dictating what is consumed for a pre-event meal. Although many commercial products provide the benefit of convenience, there are no magical foods or products that will improve the performance of all athletes.

Carbohydrate Loading

Carbohydrate loading, also known as glycogen loading, has been shown to provide an advantage for performance for some athletes participating in prolonged endurance events. As the name implies, carbohydrate loading is a process whereby the athlete consumes high levels of carbohydrates in the days preceding an event. These extra carbohydrates maximize the storage of carbohydrates (glycogen) in the muscle and liver. A recommended technique for achieving the goal of loading the muscle and liver with glycogen includes tapering the volume of exercise 6 days preceding the event. At this time, carbohydrate intake should comprise approximately 70% of the energy in the diet. Caloric restriction is not recommended during this period, since the total grams of carbohydrate would likely be diminished and glycogen storage would be decreased.

Studies have shown that carbohydrate loading can be effective in prolonging endurance in events lasting at least 90 minutes or of events that are intermittent in nature and performed at very high intensities. Athletes should experiment to determine if carbohydrate loading works for their particular sport. Some athletes have noted some minor side effects that can be either unpleasant or may impair performance. These include gastrointestinal discomfort, weight gain, sluggishness, cramping, and related effects. Weight gain occurs due to increased retention of water that is stored along with the glycogen. Additionally, though no research exists on carbohydrate loading in bodybuilders, some athletes have claimed that the extra water increases muscle volume, providing a larger appearance. Others have suggested that the water retention can cause the muscles to appear less defined. Individual athletes should decide whether or not carbohydrate loading is beneficial or detrimental. Athletic trainers must be aware of the foods and commercial products that can provide the athlete with the carbohydrates needed to achieve this level of dietary intake. In general, nutrient dense foods from the bottom three tiers of the Food Guide Pyramid should be the focus of dietary intake during carbohydrate loading. Table 13-2 provides a list of a few rich sources of carbohydrates that can be incorporated into the athlete's diet.

Age and Gender Differences

The basic recommendations for dietary intake presented previously cross age and gender boundaries for most athletes. There are, however, a few important considerations regarding age and gender that are worth mentioning.

The Food Guide Pyramid is currently recommended for anyone 2 years of age or older. This can certainly serve as the basis for recommendations for athletes of all ages. Athletic trainers working with young athletes should keep in mind the importance of adequate calories and protein for optimal promotion of growth. Dietary restriction for weight loss or maintenance is generally not recommended for young athletes unless excess weight should be lost due to health problems. Overall, the dietary goals of young athletes should be to provide adequate energy, fluid, and nutrients to optimize growth while enhancing performance.

Dietary recommendations for older athletes should also include the Food Guide Pyramid. Although aging may alter metabolism to some degree, a natural varied diet remains the basis for good health and performance. Research indicates that athletic trainers may want to pay

Table 13-2

FOODS AND SPORTS PRODUCTS RICH IN CARBOHYDRATES AND LOW IN FAT

Bread, Cereal, Rice and Pasta Group
Whole wheat bread or toast
White bread or toast
Bagels
English muffins
Flour tortillas
Corn tortillas
Crackers
Pretzels
Pancakes and waffles
Cooked cereal
Ready-to-eat cereal
Brown rice
White rice
Pasta
Noodles
Others

Vegetable Group
Corn
Peas
Potatoes
Sweet potatoes
Others (many others have few overall calories)

Fruit Group
Raw fruits
Canned fruits
Dried fruits
Fruit juices
Fruit smoothies

Milk, Yogurt, and Cheese Group
Skim milk
Low-fat ice cream/Ice milk
Low or non-fat yogurt
Fat free cheese

Meat, Poultry, Fish, Dry Beans, Eggs, and Nuts Group
Dry beans
Lentils

Table 13-2 continued

Chestnuts
Sweets (usually low nutrient density)
Low-fat cookies, snacks and desserts
Table sugar
Candy
Soft-drinks
Jam/jelly
Honey
Syrup
Sports products (usually low nutrient density)
Sports drinks
High carbohydrate sports drinks
Sports bars
Sports gels

closer attention to intake of adequate amounts of fluid, calcium, vitamin D, vitamin B6, and vitamin B12.

Female athletes tend to have more difficulty obtaining adequate nutrient intake than male athletes. Nutrients of greatest concern for the female athlete include calcium and iron; however, studies also indicate that women may also be at increased risk for dietary deficiency of energy, protein, and zinc. The athletic trainer should stress the importance of these nutrients for maximizing health and performance for his/her female athletes. The athletic trainer should emphasize that adequate consumption of these nutrients is possible through eating wholesome foods.

Weight-Conscious Athletes

Many athletes are concerned about losing weight or maintaining a low weight for competition. For example, wrestlers, boxers, rowers, and other athletes often compete in events in which there are specified weight classes that cannot be exceeded for participation. Other athletes, such as gymnasts, ballet dancers, and bodybuilders participate in sports in which they are judged on aesthetics in movement and form. Many of these athletes are often concerned about their weight, are more likely to have nutritional inadequacies, and may be predisposed to eating disorders (ie, anorexia nervosa and bulimia nervosa).

The basic diet for a weight-conscious athlete should be no different than that described previously. A diet based on the Food Guide Pyramid should provide all of the nutrients needed to allow the athlete to perform optimally. Studies suggest, however, that these athletes are less likely than other athletes to consume an adequate diet. To maximize performance, athletic trainers should pay close attention to the dietary practices of these athletes. Additionally, the athletic trainer should be aware of warning signs that can indicate that the athlete may be suffering from an eating disorder. Although eating disorders are more prevalent in these weight-conscious athletes, the athletic trainer should keep in mind that eating disorders also occur in other types of athletes as well.

Eating disorders are extremely complex in nature. Symptoms vary with the disorder but often include 1) low body weight, 2) being overly concerned about body weight or having a fear of fatness, 3) having a distorted body image, 4) having abnormal eating habits which may include restrained eating, binge eating, or purging, 5) preoccupation with food, and/or 6) abnormal or loss of menstruation.

Although disordered eating can devastate athletic performance, effects on health can be much more severe. Athletic trainers should be knowledgeable of the local resources available to athletes who may have an eating disorder. Team physicians, registered dietitians, college or university health programs, and community eating disorder programs can all be used as references by the athletic trainer. Treatment usually requires a team approach including the services of a physician, psychologist, dietitian, and possibly other healthcare workers. The presence of eating disorders, and their relationship to the "female athlete triad" are discussed in Chapter 12, Special Populations.

Chapter Fourteen

Current Knowledge of Supplements for Strength or Endurance

Mark Kern, PhD, RD

PREVALENCE OF SUPPLEMENT USE IN ATHLETES

Athletes are constantly searching for a special food or dietary supplement that will give them an advantage over the competition. Substances that provide such an advantage are referred to as ergogenic aids, meaning that they enhance performance. It's no surprise that manufacturers of these products often market their goods with the athlete in mind. A 1993 survey of five magazines containing advertisements for products marketed toward body-building athletes showed that at least 624 products were available and over 800 claims of performance enhancement with the use of these products were made. The majority of the claims made were not substantiated by research.

Each year athletes and sports teams spend millions of dollars on questionable products marketed to enhance performance. Athletic trainers are often responsible for providing athletes with accurate information regarding the use of these products, which more often than not, do not "live up" to their claims. For many products, research on their efficacy is often unavailable, deficient in proper study design, or provides no evidence of benefit; however, research on some products generally indicates that a few purported ergogenic aids may improve performance.

COMMON SUPPLEMENTS

The term "ergogenic aid" can be very misleading. One often perceives a compound called an ergogenic aid as a product that is sure to improve performance. In reality, this term is used to describe both effective and ineffective supplements marketed to improve performance. More accurate terminology for unproven products is needed to avoid confusing questionable products with substances for which there is good scientific basis to believe that improvements in performance are truly possible. A better term that more accurately reflects the dubious nature of unproven products is "ergogenic prospect." This terminology neither suggests that a product is effective or ineffective, but rather describes a product for which there is not enough high-quality scientific research to suggest that the product is truly ergogenic. The term can also be used when referring to the use of a known ergogenic aid for a purpose in which there is an absence of research that demonstrates positive effects. For example, many researchers regard creatine as an ergogenic aid for repetitive high-intensity exercise bouts. However, it is not known to be effective in improving endurance; thus for repetitive sprints it may accurately be called an ergogenic aid, but for endurance events it should be considered an ergogenic prospect.

Tables 14-1 and 14-2 provide lists of several ergogenic aids and ergogenic prospects, common claims made by their manufacturers, and a very brief summary of the research related to the product. These tables represent a fraction of the products available to athletes and the claims made for their use. Additionally, the summary of research provides an overall guide to help the athletic trainer and athlete decide if a supplement may be of benefit and does not necessarily represent the outcome of all studies on the compounds.

TIPS FOR EVALUATING SUPPLEMENT CLAIMS

New products are continually made available to consumers. Additionally, more research on nutritional ergogenic aids and prospects is being added to the base of scientific literature. Sifting through evidence to decide whether or not to recommend consumption of an ergogenic prospect can be time-consuming and difficult. Athletic trainers should consider the following simple tips when evaluating the claims for use of specific ergogenic prospects.

1) Ask yourself if the claim sounds too good to be true. If so, it almost surely is.
2) Don't rely on testimonials from famous athletes. Recognize the potential biases of those being paid to promote a product. Remember that positive effects reported for an individual or two does not establish efficacy.
3) Beware of literature provided by manufacturers. Most often this information has not undergone scrutiny of experts in the field of sports nutrition and usually provides a biased view of the product.
4) Determine if the claim is based on sound scientific research.

To fully evaluate the potential efficacy of an ergogenic prospect, the athletic trainer must be willing to investigate the evidence provided through research published in peer-reviewed journals such as the *International Journal of Sport Nutrition, Medicine and Science in Sports and Exercise*, and many other well-respected journals. Publication in such a journal should not be interpreted to indicate fact; however, evidence obtained from a source other than a peer-reviewed journal should be reviewed with even greater caution. Butterfield recently presented a summary of criteria that can be used to evaluate journal articles. Briefly, key considerations include the experience and reputation of the author(s), a well-justified research design and methodology including appropriate scientific control, and complete and clear results that are properly interpreted with no speculation of their significance.

Information about many questionable products can be obtained from the National Council for Reliable Health Information (NCRHI), formally known as the National Council Against Health Fraud (NCAHF). The NCRHI can be accessed via the Internet at www.ncahf.org. Reviews of all ineffective or potentially hazardous products are not available through the NCRHI. Other potential sources of accurate, up-to-date information include registered dietitians, physicians, peer-reviewed journals, and books written by reputable authors in the area of sports nutrition. Additionally, valuable information can be obtained from published guidelines and Internet websites of scientifically based organizations such as the American Dietetic Association and its practice group known as Sports, Cardiovascular and Wellness Nutritionists, the American College of Sports Medicine, the American Society for Nutritional Sciences, the American Medical Association, the Food and Drug Administration, the Department of Health and Human Services, the National Institutes of Health, and other highly recognized organizations.

To keep informed of the latest supplements and claims that athletes may come across, visiting local nutrition shops or health food stores and periodically reviewing popular sports magazines may be valuable to the athletic trainer. Perusing store shelves and speaking with the employees can provide tremendous insight into the tactics used to convince an athlete to use a supplement. An awareness of what is available to the athlete will provide the athletic trainer with knowledge about products prior to being asked about them by the athlete. This may give the athletic trainer an advantage in either recommending the product or suggesting to the athlete that purchasing the product is most likely a waste of money. Remember that it is probably easier to prevent an athlete from starting to use an ineffective product than to convince him/her to discontinue using a supplement that he/she is already consuming.

CONSIDERATIONS IN DISCUSSING SUPPLEMENTS WITH ATHLETES

Without a doubt certain nutritional practices can contribute to the success of an athlete. Even when considering supplements for which little or no current research suggests a beneficial effect, there is the possibility of a real physiological or pharmacological effect that may be specific to the individual or sport in which he/she is participating, or there may be some positive psychological benefit. Alternatively, cons of using a particular supplement may include excessive expense, a false sense of security, side effects, or illegality. The challenge for an athletic trainer is to provide the athlete with the necessary information so that he/she can put the athletic trainers' knowledge into practice and make an informed decision on using the product. Athletic trainers should always consider the following three issues when assisting athletes with the use of nutritional products: 1) legal concerns, 2) health risks, and 3) maintaining rapport with the athlete.

From a legal perspective, athletic trainers should recommend that athletes abstain from all substances banned for use during competition or considered illegal by state or federal laws. Though some of these substances can improve performance, legal and health complications

Table 14-1

COMMON ERGOGENIC AIDS AND ERGOGENIC PROSPECTS MARKETED FOR STRENGTH, MUSCLE BUILDING, SPEED, AND WEIGHT LOSS

Compound	Common Claim	Research Findings
Protein powder	Muscle building, strength	no benefit over dietary protein
Arginine, lysine, ornithine	Muscle building, strength	not supported by research
Creatine	Speed, increased lean weight, strength	overall supported by research
Inosine	Strength	not supported by research
Yohimbine	Muscle building, strength	not supported by research
Glandulars	Muscle building, strength	not supported by research
Vitamin B12	Muscle building	not supported by research
Antioxidant vitamins	Decrease muscle damage	more research needed
Carnitine	Fat loss	not supported by research
Chromium	Muscle building, fat loss	overall not supported by research
Boron	Muscle building, strength	not supported by research
Magnesium	Strength	preliminary support by research
Zinc	Strength	preliminary support by research
Omega-3 Fatty acids	Muscle building, strength	not supported by research
Gamma oryzanol	Muscle building, strength	not supported by research
Smilax	Muscle building, strength	not supported by research
Hydroxy methyl butyrate(HMB)	Muscle building, strength	not supported by research
Glycine	muscle building, strength	not supported by research

Table 14-2

COMMON ERGOGENIC AIDS AND ERGOGENIC PROSPECTS MARKETED WITH CLAIMS FOR ENHANCED ENDURANCE

Compound	Research Findings
Bee Pollen	not supported by research
Brewer's Yeast	not supported by research
Carnitine	overall not supported by research
Choline	more research is needed
Ginseng	not supported by research
Octacosanol	not supported by research
Pangamic acid	not supported by research
Medium Chain Triglycerides	more research is needed
Branched Chain Amino Acids	overall not supported by research
Caffeine	overall supported by research
Coenzyme Q	not supported by research
Tryptophan	not supported by research
Aspartate salts	more research is needed
Dihydroxyacetone and pyruvate	preliminary: supported by research
Lactate	not supported by research
Spirulina	not supported by research
Inosine	not supported by research
Glutamine	not supported by research
Glycerol	more research is needed
Wheat germ oil	not supported by research

far outweigh their benefits. For ergogenic aids and prospects that are illegal only if a certain threshold of consumption is surpassed, such as caffeine, the athletic trainer must provide guidance for the maximum recommended level of intake. Athletic trainers should remain up-to-date on which substances are banned and which products include those substances. Some products may include a banned substance, yet be marketed for containing another. For example, some brands of aspirin also contain caffeine. An athlete using such a product must be careful not to exceed the maximum legal intake of the banned substance to avoid risk disqualification or worse.

For substances that are not banned, health risks may still be an important issue. Many products marketed as ergogenic aids possess health risks and are often not regulated by the FDA. Athletes often make the mistake of assuming that since a product is available for purchase it must be safe and effective. In reality, numerous products are known to potentially cause a variety of health problems, and other products often lack research on short-term and/or long-term health implications. When it comes to dietary supplements, the common phrase "buyer beware" is extremely appropriate. Each athlete has the right to weigh the potential benefits versus potential side-effects in making his/her decision about using a supplement; however, the athletic trainer can often provide valuable information that will allow the athlete to make the best choice.

In addition to having a direct impact on health status, some products may have hazardous effects by replacing natural, wholesome food. The product selected may not provide the same nutrients that would be obtained through the food the athlete has given up in favor of the supplement. Overuse of such products may lead to a nutritional inadequacy that could impair performance and/or adversely affect health. In this way, the product itself is not causing harm, but it is still producing a damaging outcome.

As described by Butterfield, maintaining rapport with an athlete who is using a questionable ergogenic prospect that lacks evidence for efficacy, but appears to be safe, can be very important. A good relationship with the athlete may allow the athletic trainer to provide valuable assistance that may otherwise be dismissed in the absence of such rapport. Rapport can be lost when the athletic trainer tells an athlete that he/she will obtain no benefit from a product that the athlete believes will work. Athletic trainers should keep in mind that some athletes are prone to the "placebo effect." These athletes may obtain benefit from a product simply by believing it will work. Additionally, many athletes are sponsored by manufacturers of questionable products. Recommending that the athlete not use a product provided by a sponsor may strain the relationship between the athletic trainer and athlete. Furthermore, many times coaches or teammates suggest using specific compounds. Under such circumstances, allowing the use of safe ergogenic prospects is warranted to prevent problems for the athlete, team, or athletic trainer. As stated by Butterfield, "…this year's ergogenic aid is next year's garbage," so if there are valid reasons to allow an athlete to use a questionable product that is considered safe, such use will often be short-lived and without incident.

Overall, proper nutrition can prevent performance decrements that occur with nutritional deficiencies or excesses. Athletic trainers should attempt to instill in their athletes the idea that following good dietary practices is an important component of an optimal training regimen. Athletes should follow basic dietary guidelines stressing a diet high in carbohydrates and fluids to ensure adequate intake of energy, nutrients and water. Athletic trainers may wish to encourage athletes to consult a registered dietitian for professional help in regard to proper dietary intake. Furthermore, athletic trainers should keep in mind that although evidence suggests that a few dietary practices may enhance performance, most nutritional ergogenic prospects are marketed without scientific research that demonstrates efficacy. These products should be used only after considering safety and legality.

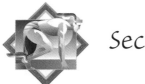

Section 5

Injury Prevention and Management Techniques

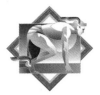

Chapter Fifteen

Flexibility Training

Flexibility is the ability of a joint to move throughout the range of motion (ROM). Flexibility training should be an important part of an athlete's training program. Regardless of the sport in which the athlete is active, flexibility training can lead to improved performance, quicker recovery time between exercise sessions, and injury prevention. Even greater emphasis should be placed on flexibility training in the elderly population. Some of the physiological changes occurring with age, outlined in the previous chapters, also lead to a decline in musculoskeletal flexibility. It is also well known that men tend to be less flexible than women. Specifically when it comes to the prevention of low back pain, you should include flexibility exercises for the low back, hamstrings, and hip flexors. Flexibility is dependent upon the congenital structure of the joint, distensibility of the joint capsule, previous injury or surgery involving a joint, amount of adipose tissue or muscle mass (which if excessive can restrict movement), muscle temperature and extensibility of muscles, tendons, ligaments, and fascia. Flexibility can be measured using a goniometer device, Leighton flexometer, or by performing simple tasks that serve as flexibility screening tools. Encourage your athletes to include flexibility training as part of their warm-up and cool-down periods, with an emphasis placed on the cool-down period when body temperature is elevated and muscles are pliable. Even during the warm-up period, it is recommended that athletes precede stretching with a brief bout of aerobic activity that increases their heart rate and muscle temperature.

There are basically three types of flexibility training: static, dynamic (ballistic), and proprioceptive neuromuscular facilitation (PNF). Each type of training is targeted at elongation of the muscles and tendons. More advanced joint mobilization techniques are needed for ligamentous, capsular, or bony changes in ROM and need to be performed by a trained clinician. Static and dynamic stretching can be performed as an individual or in a group, as PNF stretching requires the use of a knowledgeable partner, athletic trainer, or strength and conditioning specialist.

STATIC STRETCHING

Static stretching occurs when the athlete gradually moves the limb or body area through a ROM and holds the motion at the end range for a period of time. For example, a static hamstring stretch is performed by having an athlete sit with both legs extended in front of him/her and slowly reach for his/her ankles while keeping the back straight until tension is felt at the end ROM; then hold this position for 10 to 15 seconds. One modification to this technique is to incorporate active contraction of the quadriceps muscle group in order to elicit a greater relaxation response in the antagonist muscle group (hamstrings). In order to optimize elongation of the muscle group, the stretch position for each muscle group is usually repeated three times with rest periods in between. If the athlete is trying to improve flexibility following immobilization, surgery, and/or injury, a longer duration stretch-hold (30 to 60 seconds) and up to five repetitions are recommended. Keep in mind that the stretch intensity should be performed to the point of muscle tension, but never to the point of pain. Normal flexibility training need only occur before and after the exercise activity. If improvements in flexibility are being targeted, you should perform the flexibility exercises several times a day.

DYNAMIC STRETCHING

If the same exercise is performed but the stretch consists of a series of bouncing movements in an attempt to reach further with each bounce, then a dynamic stretch of the hamstrings is being performed. Dynamic or ballistic stretching is rarely prescribed anymore because it has been shown to contribute to the increased risk of injury and muscle soreness, especially when the bouncing movements are extreme. If a muscle is stretching too quickly or in a jerky fashion, then the body responds with a stretch reflex, which is a protective mechanism that results in contraction of the muscle being stretched. Not only is this contrary to what the athlete is trying to accomplish but can also lead to excessive muscle soreness and possibly musculoskeletal injury. The mechanisms of the stretch reflex are addressed in detail in Chapter Six.

PROPRIOCEPTIVE NEUROMUSCULAR FACILITATION

PNF stretching was introduced in the late 1950s and is based upon neuromuscular principles centered on the action of the Golgi Tendon Organ (GTO) and muscle spindle; and mechanical aspects of the muscle itself. The GTO is located in the musculotendinous region of the muscle and is responsible for sensing tension in the muscle. It serves as a protective mechanism in that when the tension is too great, an inhibitory reflex occurs, causing the muscle to relax. The muscle spindle is located throughout the muscle itself and is positioned parallel to the muscle fibers. The muscle spindle senses changes in the length of the muscle. If the change in length is too abrupt, the muscle spindle can overfire, resulting in a muscle spasm and may indirectly lead to spasticity. During PNF stretching, the GTO comes into play when the muscle is in spasm or is spastic. If a spastic muscle, or one that is in spasm, contracts, the GTO fires, and as a result, autogenically inhibits the contracting muscle. This mechanism occurs as a result of inhibition of the muscle spindle in that particular muscle. Fatigue occurs by contracting the muscle for approximately 5 seconds. Therefore, inhibition of the muscle spindle and fatigue both contribute to relaxation of a spastic muscle or one that is in spasm.

Another mechanism by which PNF stretching optimizes muscle length involves the mechanical components of the muscle. The neurological effects of PNF stretching described above would not play a significant role in stretching the muscles of a healthy athlete who does not have muscles that are in spasm. In this case, when a tight muscle contracts isometrically, the sarcomere shortens, thereby causing passive elongation of the muscle connective tissue and tendons. The muscle is in a sense mechanically stretching itself. Fatigue also plays a role in healthy muscles and contributes to relaxation of the muscle and, ultimately elongation. There are two different PNF stretching techniques; contract-relax and hold-relax.

Contract-Relax

The contract-relax technique involves a series of active muscle contractions followed by relaxation. The goal of this technique is to increase active range of motion in the absence of pain. The key component to the contract-relax technique is to allow for some movement, specifically rotational movement during the contraction phase of the technique. During the relaxation phase it is advised that the athlete actively move the joint further through the range of motion, optimizing elongation of the muscle. The following example is given for stretching the hamstring muscle group.

With the athlete lying supine, he/she actively moves the hip of one leg into flexion, slight abduction, and internal rotation while keeping the knee extended until maximum tension is developed. The partner or athletic trainer is present and guides the athlete through this motion. The partner could also passively move the hip into this position if the athlete is unfamiliar with the movement pattern or unable to properly perform the movement.

The partner then asks the athlete to push down isometrically while externally rotating the hip. The contraction should be strong and smooth and performed with increasing intensity against the partner's resistance until maximum force is developed. The partner should allow for slight movement, especially the rotational movement, of the lower limb to be sure all muscles are contracting. The athlete holds the contraction for 5 seconds, then relaxes the muscle gradually.

After the athlete relaxes the hamstring muscle group, the athlete repositions the hip into a greater degree of hip flexion. The partner should again guide this motion and may even reposition the hip passively.

Hold-Relax

The hold-relax technique is essentially the same as the contract-relax technique, but no movement is allowed during the contraction phase. The goal of this technique is to also increase active range of motion, but it may also be used in treating pain caused by a restricted muscle. The hamstring muscles are again used as an example of this technique.

With the athlete lying supine, he/she actively moves the hip of one leg into flexion, slight abduction, and internal rotation while keeping the knee extended until maximum tension is developed. The partner or athletic trainer is present and guides the athlete through this motion. The partner could also passively move the hip into this position if the athlete is unfamiliar with the movement pattern or unable to properly perform the movement.

The athlete is then asked to perform an isometric contraction against the partner's resistance. The contraction should be performed gradually until maximum tension is developed. Instruct the athlete to attempt to move the leg down and in, while rotating the leg outward. The athlete holds this contraction for 5 seconds, then is instructed to slowly relax. Again, it is important during this technique not to allow for any movement during the contraction or hold phase.

Once fully relaxed, the athlete then actively repositions the leg into further hip flexion while the partner guides the athlete through this motion. The partner may also reposition the hip passively.

Each stretch should be repeated several times to optimize flexibility in the muscles. If the partner is passively repositioning the joint, care should be taken not to stretch the hamstrings too far. If the athletic trainer or another capable partner is not available, the athlete may use a door jam to support the leg, then move his/her body forward to move the hip through the ROM.

Studies examining all three types of flexibility training have reported contradicting evidence for the support of one method over another. In general, static stretching is recommended for individual use and group-led warm-up and cool-down activities. PNF techniques require the use of a knowledgeable partner and are more complicated to perform. PNF should be used to meet the needs of certain sports in which injury rates are high in particular muscle groups; they are also prescribed for individual athletes following injury as part of a comprehensive injury rehabilitation program. When performing any type of flexibility exercise, body position, posture, and technique of performance are critical to the success of the exercise. As an athletic trainer, it is your job to educate athletes about the proper techniques of flexibility training.

INJURY PREVENTION TECHNIQUES

The following stretching techniques are recommended for each injury condition and should be performed bilaterally, where appropriate. It is beyond the scope of this text to incorporate all sport injuries. The more common ailments, however, are included.

Low Back Pain

HIP FLEXOR STRETCH

Position feet together, hands on hips, and feet facing forward. With one foot, step forward keeping the pelvis tucked under your body, and direct the opposite knee toward the ground into a lunge position. This is the hip flexor that is being stretched. Be careful not to allow the front knee to protrude past the toes. If this occurs, take a bigger step and maintain the knee over the toes.

SUPINE HAMSTRING STRETCH

Lie supine with one leg extended in the air and held in place with both hands. Actively flex this hip with assistance from your hands, pulling your leg back toward you. The opposite hip and knee are flexed with the foot positioned on the ground. Your neck and shoulders should be relaxed.

HAMSTRING STRETCH

In a sitting position, place one leg in front of you on the floor with the knee extended. Be sure the toes are pointed upward with the tibia positioned in a neutral position. The opposite leg should be positioned in a figure-four position with the sole of the foot resting next to the inside portion of the thigh of the extended leg. Keeping the back extended, reach forward with both hands toward the foot of the extended leg.

SINGLE KNEE-TO-CHEST STRETCH

Lying supine, bring one knee to your chest while keeping the other leg extended on the ground. The extended leg may also be flexed with the foot on the ground to support the low back.

LATERAL ROTATIONS

Lie supine with both hips and knees flexed. Leave both feet on the ground. Slowly, allow the knees to fall to one side with the pull of gravity. Do not accommodate the movement by rolling onto your side.

PIRIFORMIS OR LATERAL HIP STRETCH

Sitting, place the right foot over the left knee and place next to the outer thigh of the left leg. With your left arm, pull the right knee into your chest while rotating to the right.

QUADRUPED

Position the body on hands and knees. Then push the buttocks back toward the heels and stretch forward with the arms. Keep the neck relaxed.

Frozen Shoulder Syndrome

ARM IN FRONT STRETCH

Bring the arm across the chest, place the opposite hand over the elbow and pull it toward the opposite shoulder.

ARM BEHIND STRETCH

Place both arms straight up in the air over the head. Allow one elbow to flex and the forearm to fall behind the head. With the other hand, grasp the flexed elbow and pull downward behind the head.

DOUBLE CLASP STRETCH

Clasp both hands together behind you. Slowly lift both arms up toward the ceiling keeping the trunk erect and not bending forward at the hips.

CORNER WALL STRETCH

Face forward in a corner, placing one hand on each wall of the corner with the elbows extended. With the feet together and away from the corner, lean into the corner, allowing the elbows to bend until a gentle stretch is perceived.

Carpal Tunnel Syndrome

PALM STRETCH

Place the palms of both hands together in a praying position. Slowly extend the wrists by pushing downward keeping the palms together and in front of you.

WRIST EXTENSION STRETCH

Grab the palm of one hand, extend your elbows, keeping the bottom forearm supinated. Slowly extend the wrist by pulling it downward toward your body.

Achilles-Tightness

STRAIGHT LEG STRETCH

Stand against the wall with the target leg extended back away from the wall. While keeping the heel on the ground, lean forward into the wall until tension is felt in the achilles tendon. If you do not perceive tension, move the foot farther away from the wall.

BENT KNEE STRETCH

Position yourself as if performing the straight leg stretch, only bend slightly at the knee and lean forward into the wall.

PLATFORM STRETCH

Using a slanted platform, stand with your knee extended and the heel positioned further down on the slope and allow the achilles tendon to stretch. Repeat the stretch with the knee slightly flexed.

(Note: With any of the achilles stretches, you can also internally and externally rotate your foot to emphasize the stretch medially or laterally.)

Iliotibial Band Tightness

CROSSOVER STRETCH

Standing, place the right foot over the left, crossing at the knees. Allow the knees to bend slightly, then bend forward at the waist and reach for the floor. Rotate slightly to the left, allowing the right hip to jut outward, targeting a lateral hip stretch.

SITTING LATERAL HIP STRETCH

Sitting, place the right foot over the left knee and place next to the outer thigh of the left leg. With your left arm, pull the right knee into your chest while rotating to the right.

SUPINE LATERAL HIP STRETCH

Lying supine, cross your knees, keeping the bottom foot on the ground. Allow your legs to fall to the side of the top leg, stretching your opposite hip.

SIDEWAY WALL STRETCH

Stand with your left hip facing a wall and place your left hand up on the wall for support. Cross your right foot over your left foot, crossing at the knees. Lean into the wall by protruding your left hip toward the wall.

DOORWAY STRETCH

Lie supine in a doorway. Flex your hip and position it across your body, keeping your knee extended. Place your heel on the wall and stretch your lateral hip.

FIGURE-FOUR STRETCH

Stand in front of a table or ledge. Place your lower leg and foot up on the table or ledge so it is parallel with the ground, then lean forward into your leg, placing a stretch on your lateral hip.

Plantar Facitis

ACHILLES STRETCHES

Described above.

PASSIVE ANKLE DORSIFLEXION AND TOE EXTENSION STRETCH

This stretch can be performed individually or by a partner. Passively dorsiflex your ankle while simultaneously extending your toes backward as far as possible.

BOTTLE STRETCH

Using a bottle or other cylindrical object, roll the object under the sole of your foot while dorsiflexing your ankle and extending your toes. Move your foot back and forth over the object. Using a water bottle filled with frozen water allows you to perform the exercise while applying ice to the area.

USEFUL RESOURCES

There are multitudes of references available on flexibility training exercises. In particular, *Stretching* by Bob Anderson and the PNF textbook by Sue Adlers listed in the Bibliography list, are especially useful. Flexibility exercises should be prescribed individually for each sport. The muscles used in different sports vary and care should be taken in adapting certain stretching exercises to meet the needs and demands of each sport. Stretches specific to a particular movement or sport are known as functional stretches. For example, a baseball player performs functional stretches when he/she uses the bat to move through the swinging motion at a slow-controlled pace. Similarly, a golfer uses a golf club to stretch the muscles used during a golf swing. A swimmer might mimic the motion of a particular stroke, emphasizing slow, controlled movement with elongation of the muscle at the end range of motion. Regardless of the sport or activity, be sure to encourage all athletes to incorporate a sound, sport-specific stretching program.

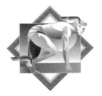

Chapter Sixteen

Special Concerns

INJURY MANAGEMENT TECHNIQUES

Knowledge is the key to successful injury prevention and management. Injury management is imperative to quicken recovery and minimize time lost from activity. The back stabilization, hip, abdominal, rotator cuff, and rice routines in Chapter Seventeen are good programs to implement into a rehabilitation or management plan as indicated. The upper and lower extremity plyometrics and maintenance weightlifting programs are also recommended during the last phase of rehabilitation or injury management, as the athlete progresses back into full play. This section will discuss the appropriate techniques required, regardless of age and experience, to help reduce the probability of a debilitating injury.

BREATHING TECHNIQUES

When executing strength training techniques it is very important to breathe and breathe correctly. For low to moderate intensities, holding the breath during the execution and/or return phase may be very dangerous in that the brain is being deprived of oxygen, which in turn may cause dizziness. For example, during the power squat exercise, inhalation occurs in the return phase as the body descends into the squat position. The execution phase is the ascension from squat to upright position, in which exhalation occurs.

When high intensities and low volume are required, or when executing power-lifting techniques, breathing modification must take place. Prior to the execution phase, a deeper breath is inhaled and held until the sticking point has been reached. Exhalation then occurs and a few breaths are taken before the next repetition is executed. Again, using the power squat exercise, inhalation occurs while descending or during the return phase. As ascension is initiated, the breath is held and exhaled once the upright position has been achieved.

Executing Olympic lifting techniques, such as the power clean, requires yet another method of breathing. The use of multiple breaths during one repetition is necessary. As the barbell leaves the ground during the first pull, the lifter inhales. When the lifter executes the second pull, as the bar passes the knees, he/she exhales. Once the bar is caught and begins to lower to the knees, inhalation occurs. From the knees to the floor, the lifter exhales.

GRIP AND PLACEMENT

The choice of grip and its width on the weight or apparatus is dependent on not only what exercise is being executed but also on the desired involvement of specific muscles. For example, performing a pull-up with an overhand or pronated grip will emphasize the muscles of the back, whereas a reverse or supinated grip will initiate the biceps brachii. The overhand is the more commonly used grip in Power and Olympic lifting. However, someone performing the dead lift could use the overhand or alternating grip. The alternating grip has both thumbs pointing in the same direction, one hand is overhand, and the other is reversed. Regardless of the grip choice and width placement, a closed grip is mandatory as opposed to an open grip in which the thumb does not wrap around the bar or apparatus. The chance of losing the bar during a lift decreases with the closed grip.

MOVING THE WEIGHT FROM THE GROUND

When initiating a lift or picking a weight up correctly, important elements must be maintained each and every time. Starting from the ground up, the feet, placed shoulder width apart or more, must remain flat with the toes slightly pointed outward. The wider the stance, the greater the stability and, thus, balance. This is very important when performing overhead lifting techniques. Make sure the barbell is close to the shins to ensure primary usage of the legs and not the back. While keeping elbows extended, head up, and eyes straight ahead, squat down to grip the barbell. Check to see that the grip is correct and balanced. The back is kept flat and shoulders are above the hips and over the bar. During ascension, the bar is kept very close to the body. Drive the hips and chest up while extending the legs, concentrating on contracting the glutes, quadriceps, and hamstrings. The heels never leave the ground, the hips never pass or move in front of the shoulders, the back remains flat, and the eyes continue looking forward. Teaching this technique may limit many unnecessary back injuries. Having the athlete practice in front of a mirror will provide invaluable feedback.

RETURNING THE WEIGHT TO THE GROUND

When returning the bar to the ground, emphasize the same technique as that of lifting the bar from the ground, only in reverse. Keep the body weight on the heels, back flat, head and chest up, shoulders above hips, and eyes looking forward. Still keeping the weight close to the body, stress a slow and controlled descent. If the weight is held overhead, allow the weight to lower to the thighs with hips and knees slightly flexed before moving it to the floor.

SPOTTING RECOMMENDATIONS

The responsibilities of the spotter regarding safety issues were emphasized in Chapter Two. The following are some recommendations for the attentive spotter:

- Ensure the lifting area is free of debris.
- Communicate with the lifter on how many repetitions are being attempted and when assistance is usually required.
- Check to see that the barbell is loaded appropriately and evenly and that the correct grip is being used.
- Pay attention to the lifter and do not become distracted from the area or the number of repetitions.
- Be in correct position to assist so you (the spotter) do not sustain injury. Keep knees and hips slightly flexed and back flat.
- Your hands should be close to the bar without obstructing the lifter's movement or vision.
- Know the correct technique of the lift and the path the weight should travel.
- Know your (the spotter's) limitations. Do not attempt to spot a weight that is beyond what you can handle.
- Incorporate the use of another spotter for Power lifts, one on each end if the weight is excessive.
- Suggest any form changes to ensure proper strength-training techniques.

POWER LIFTING

Once the athlete has been instructed on techniques of the bench press, dead lift, and squat (see weightlifting descriptions for details), there are some points that should be continually observed and emphasized by both lifter and spotter before and during the exercise.

Bench Press

- Feet flat and kept on the floor.
- Head, shoulders, and buttocks remain on the bench.
- Lumbar arch is allowed, but only if buttock remains on bench.
- Closed grip is used.
- Spotter stands behind the bench at the head of the lifter.
- The rack is at an appropriate height for safe usage.
- Spotter is used for un-racking and re-racking the bar.
- Proper breathing technique.

Dead Lift

- Feet flat and shoulder width apart.
- Barbell close to shins prior to lifting.
- Same technique as picking the weight up off the ground.
- Proper breathing technique.
- Spotter is not used for this exercise.

Squat

- Feet flat and shoulder width apart.
- Barbell is either on the anterior (front squat) or posterior (power squat) deltoids.
- Spotter stands behind the lifter and assists at the waist.
- Usage of spotting bars is suggested for heavy weights (bars are placed between uprights in the squat rack to prevent weight from falling/moving beyond a desired height).
- Proper breathing technique.

OLYMPIC LIFTING

The Olympic lifts are more challenging and will take the athlete longer to master. The spotter is positioned behind the lifter, but it is suggested that the lifter push the bar away, out in front, if the lift is going to be lost. We will analyze the two pulls involved in Olympic lifting and provide suggestions for teaching the segments.

Other than hang snatch and hang clean, the first pull comes from the ground. The same technique is used as mentioned in the section on how to pick the weight up off the floor. The second pull is from knees to shoulders or above the shoulders. The goal of these lifts is to increase power, so the weight must be moved rapidly. There must be no hesitation between pulls. Due to this movement, though, technique is sometimes negatively altered. The following are some phrases you can use to make the transition from the first to the second pull smooth.

- Keep the bar close to your body (emphasize legs rather than back).
- Grip just outside the shins for clean, wide for snatch.
- Think of the arms as extended ropes holding the bar (keeping elbows extended during the pull).
- Drive (extend) the ankles, knees, and hips simultaneously as in a vertical jump (vertical movement).
- Shrug shoulders, keeping the elbows extended as you accelerate up, as the hips drive up.
- As the bar passes the hips, the elbows flex. They are wide and away from the body.
- Pull to the shoulders for clean, pull to the face for snatch (peak of pull).
- Drop the body under the bar. Flex the ankles, knees, and hips to squat as the bar is being caught.

- During a high pull, the bar is not caught, but the body is dropped underneath at the peak of the pull and the bar is brought back down to the thighs.
- The bar is caught on the shoulders for clean, with elbows flexed and pointing forward, upper arms are parallel with the ground. The bar is caught above the head for snatch, with elbows extended.
- As the catch occurs, the body is in a squat position.
- Holding the catch, stand upright, inhale and exhale, bring the bar to the thighs then ground.

COMMON OVERUSE INJURIES

We have emphasized the importance of balancing an athlete's training schedule with the proper intensity, frequency, duration, and rate of progression. Additionally, we have provided specific strength training programs that target susceptible muscle groups. The importance of incorporating these programs into your athlete's training regimes cannot be overlooked, especially when it comes to the prevention of overuse injuries. Improper prescription and inadequate supervision of exercise training can lead to overtraining, which will invariably lead to musculoskeletal injury. Overtraining is defined as an imbalance between training and recovery. When sufficient rest is not allowed following physical activity, the body is unable to adapt to the physiological stresses placed upon musculoskeletal structures. This phenomenon is further compromised when an athlete begins an exercise training program without building baseline strength, endurance, and flexibility. The body is forced to adapt to stresses that are beyond its capabilities. It is particularly important to include trunk and hip stabilization routines as part of any athlete's introductory training period prior to intense exercise training.

Muscle imbalances, congenital abnormalities, and training errors also contribute to the incidence of overuse injuries. While little may be done about congenital abnormalities, preparticipation screening can aid in detecting muscle imbalances. Proper strength training prescription can correct muscle imbalances and may prevent future injury. Additionally, knowledge about the biomechanical aspects of a sport will aid in preventing improper training techniques that may lead to overuse injuries.

An overuse injury occurs as the result of repeated mechanical overload in which the tissue is unable to withstand or recover from the applied stresses. Stresses applied gradually over time and with the appropriate intensity allow musculoskeletal structures to adapt and strengthen. Eventually, the structures are able to tolerate greater and greater forces without incidence.

A comprehensive list of the types of overuse injuries seen with physical activity is beyond the scope of this textbook. Primarily, muscle strains, tendonitis, and stress fractures are types of musculoskeletal injuries that can be associated with most any muscle and/or joint that is overworked. Muscle strains occur when the force applied to the muscle is greater than it is able to tolerate and micro- or macrotears result. Most muscle strains occur at the musculotendinous junction, which is the weakest point of the muscle. Tendonitis, or inflammation of the tendon, is usually the result of repetitive trauma that results in irritation and/or microtears of the tendon. Stress fractures are caused by repeated stress to a bone below the fracture threshold. The most common sites for stress fractures are the metatarsals, calcaneus, and tibia. Women who are involved in the Female Athlete Triad (presented in Chapter Twelve) may be especially at risk for stress fractures due to decreased bone density levels. Regardless of the type of overuse injury, it is important to remember that most overuse injuries can be prevented through proper exercise prescription, progression, and supervision.

COMMON ACUTE INJURIES

The mechanisms of an acute injury are often less controlled than overuse injuries. However, in many instances acute injuries can be prevented. Ensuring a safe training environment is probably the number one factor in preventing acute injuries in athletes. This includes some of the safety issues discussed in Chapter Two. Keeping the training area free from debris and maintaining nonslip, even surfaces are key principles in injury prevention. Acute injuries that are the result of direct contact or immediate trauma are often not preventable, however certain steps can be taken to avoid their occurrence. For example, be sure your athletes are competing against fairly equal opponents. It is usually the smaller, younger athlete who gets injured when competing against a larger, older athlete. Also, ensuring that your athletes have baseline strength, endurance, proprioception, and flexibility may allow them to recover from an injury situation. For example, a well-trained athlete will be more likely to recover from an inversion ankle stress than a sedentary or untrained athlete. This obviously depends on the amount of stress applied, but nevertheless "an ounce of prevention is worth a pound of cure." Specific flexibility exercises for certain injury conditions are presented in Chapter Fifteen and will go a long way in not only treating but also preventing acute and chronic injuries.

Most acute injuries consist of sprains, strains, contusions, fractures, dislocations, tendon ruptures, abrasions, lacerations, avulsions, and concussions. Again, we are unable to discuss all types of acute injuries in this chapter. If you would like more information about the types of acute injuries associated with physical activity, we recommend referring to an athletic injury textbook.

Areas that are commonly injured during strength training sessions are the hips, low back, and rotator cuff. Fortunately, we have provided specific strengthening programs in Section 6 to include in the athlete's training regime. The abdominal, hip and back stabilization routines will give the lifter good core strength. The Power and Olympic lifts especially tax these areas. Prior to allowing the athlete to perform these exercises, ensure that he/she has engaged in an introductory period of strength training that includes hip, back, and abdominal work. The muscles that help stabilize a joint are usually in jeopardy of being injured because they are oftentimes not focused on during a strength training program. Therefore, we recommend that you implement the rotator cuff warm-up at the start of every strength training session. This will ready the joint surfaces and help to strengthen the small, often neglected muscles. Even the lower body sessions will utilize the shoulder girdle muscles for support.

In conclusion, take time to determine the athlete's training goals, then educate him/her on the importance of adhering to a prescribed program, and provide adequate supervision so the athlete can begin a safe and productive training program. Continue to invest time for observation and re-evaluation, and give the athlete adequate feedback so he/she may continue an effective and efficient training program.

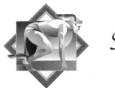

Section 6

Sport-Specific Strength
Training Programs

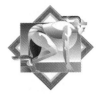

Chapter Seventeen

Supplemental Routines and Descriptions

ABDOMINAL ROUTINES AND DESCRIPTIONS

Perform exercises in the sequence in which they appear, no rest between sets. The parentheses include the number of sets and repetitions (eg, 2 x 30 means two sets of 30 repetitions).

Abdominal #1

Crunch (1 x 25): Supine, knees flexed to 90 degrees, feet on floor and arms crossed across chest. Lift shoulders off the floor. Keep the low back pushed to the floor.

Reverse crunch (1 x 25): Supine, knees flexed to 90 degrees, feet off the floor and arms at the sides. Lift the hips off the floor and crunch toward the chest. Head and shoulders remain on the floor.

Elbows and knees (1 x 25): Supine, knees flexed to 90 degrees, feet begin on the floor and hands behind the head. Lift and bring the knees and elbows together and return to the starting position.

Lying hip lift (1 x 20): Supine, hips flexed to 90 degrees, knees extended, arms at sides, head and shoulders remain on the floor. Lift hips off the floor, raising extended legs straight in the air.

Elevated leg crunch (1 x 15): Supine, knees extended, arms at the sides, lift legs 6 inches off the floor, hold and lift the shoulders off the floor. Keep feet raised during the entire set.

Sit-up (1 x 20): Supine, knees flexed, feet secure and arms crossed over chest. Raise shoulders off the floor until the elbows touch the knees.

Abdominal #2

Lateral crunch (1 x 20): Sidelying, upper arms by the ears and hands hold the opposite elbows. Keep hips and knees slightly flexed and lift the shoulder off the floor toward the hip. Continue on the same side until the set is complete.

Lateral crunch w/leg lift (1 x 10): Sidelying, upper arms by the ears and the hands hold the opposite elbows. Keep the knee slightly flexed with the top knee extended. Lift the shoulder and extended leg simultaneously. Continue on the same side until the set is complete.

Twist crunch to elbow (1 x 25): Supine, knees flexed to 90 degrees, cross one ankle on the opposing knee (foot on floor) and hands behind the head. Lift and twist the torso so the elbow reaches the opposing flexed knee. Continue on the same side until the set is complete.

Bicycle (1 x 20): Supine, hips and knees flexed, feet off the floor and hands behind the head. Twist the torso and bring together the opposing elbow and knee (for one repetition), alternate position.

Straight leg crunch (1 x 20): Supine, hips flexed to 90 degrees, knees extended and arms behind the head. Low back remains on the floor. Lift the shoulders off the floor while maintaining extended knees straight in the air.

DB side bends (1 x 20): Standing, feet shoulder width apart, knees slightly flexed, hold one dumbbell in one hand and place the other hand behind the head. Maintain stable hips and torso and lower the weight down the side toward the knee. Contract the opposite side to stand in an upright position. Continue on the same side until the set is complete.

Torso twists (1 x 20): Standing, feet shoulder width apart, knees slightly flexed, hold a wooden dowl (stick) behind the head, resting on the posterior deltoids. Twist in both directions for one repetition.

Abdominal Medicine Ball (Single)

Crunch (1 x 20): Supine, knees flexed to 90 degrees, and feet secure. Hold the medicine ball close to the chest and lift the shoulders off the floor. Keep the low back pushed to the floor. To increase difficulty, hold the medicine ball away from the body or perform on an incline bench.

Seated twist (1 x 10): Seated, knees flexed, and feet secure. Hold the medicine ball, lean back to contract the abdomen and twist in both directions for one repetition. To increase difficulty, hold the medicine ball away from the body and touch the floor or perform on an incline bench.

Seated twist release (1 x 10): Seated, knees flexed, and feet on the floor. Twist with the medicine ball and place it on the floor behind the hips. Twist to the other side and pick up the medicine ball. Continue on the same side until the set is complete.

Leg raise (1 x 10): Supine, extended knees and hands placed in the lumbar curve on the floor for support. Lift leg 6 inches to 12 inches off the floor while squeezing the medicine ball between the legs. To increase difficulty, place the ball closer to the feet.

Abdominal Medicine Ball (With Partner)

Seated crunch w/toss and catch (1 x 15): Seated, knees flexed, feet on the floor, lean back to contract the abdomen and hold the position. Toss and catch with a partner while maintaining a contracted abdomen. To increase difficulty, challenge your partner by tossing in a variety of angles.

Seated twist w/toss and catch (1 x 10): Seated, knees flexed, feet on the floor, lean back to contract the abdomen and hold the position. Twist with the medicine ball and toss it across to your partner, who catches the ball and twists to toss it. Partners will be twisting on the same side, however the ball will cross from one side to the other. Continue on the same side until the set is complete.

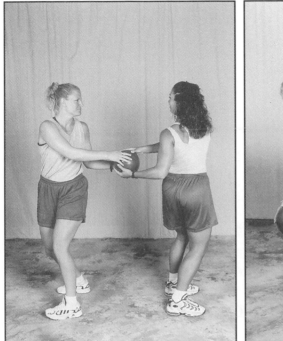

Figure 17-1. Start and finish position of a standing full twist.

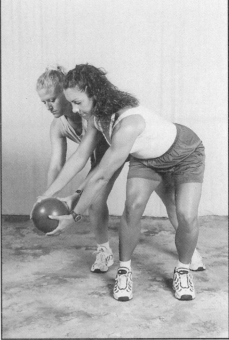

Figure 17-2a. Low point of an eccentric wood chopper.

Standing half twist (1 x 10): Standing back to back, knees slightly flexed, twist with the medicine ball and hand to your partner. Twist without the ball to the other side and retrieve it from your partner. Continue on the same side until set is complete. Partners will be twisting in opposite directions.

Standing full twist (1 x 10): Standing back to back (approximately 2 feet apart), knees slightly flexed, twist with the medicine ball and hand it to your partner. Twist without the ball to the other side and retrieve it from your partner. Continue on the same side until the set is complete. Partners will be twisting in the same directions (Figure 17-1).

Eccentric wood chopper (1 x 10): Standing, knees slightly flexed, bring the medicine ball down toward the knee, partner (standing behind) pushes at the lowest point to resist. Swing the medicine ball up over the shoulder while your partner pushes at the highest point to resist. Continue on the same side until the set is complete (Figures 17-2a, 2b).

Eccentric rotation (1x10): Standing, knees slightly flexed, rotate side to side for one repetition. Your partner stands behind and pushes at each maximal rotation point.

BACK STABILIZATION ROUTINE AND DESCRIPTION

Perform one exercise from each group for a workout routine. Increase repetitions or seconds within a set as the workout becomes easy.

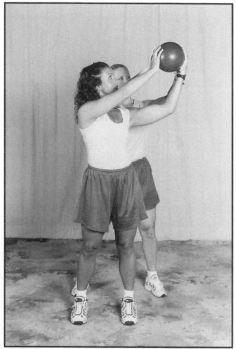

Figure 17-2b. High point of eccentric wood chopper.

Note: To find pelvic neutral: stand, kneel, sit, lie (supine or prone), or start in quadruped position. Place the hands on the ASIS (if not the quadruped). Anteriorly rotate the pelvis (forward tilt) fully, then posteriorly rotate (backward tilt) the pelvis fully. Repeat, then position the pelvis at the midrange of this motion and hold. When in neutral, the pelvis and lumbar curves are midway between a forward and backward tilt.

Group 1

Pelvic tilts (1 x 30): Supine, knees flexed to 90 degrees, feet on floor, arms at the sides and hands on the anterior superior iliac spine (ASIS). Posteriorly rotate the ASIS, contract the lower abdomen, push the low back into the floor without raising the hips. Hold for 3 seconds for one repetition.

Dead bug (1 x 15): Supine, hips and knee flexed to 90 degrees, and feet on the floor. Arms at the sides and pelvis in neutral. Without deviating pelvic or knee positions, lower one heel to the floor and return to the starting position (hip/knee at 90 degrees), then lower the opposite leg and return to the starting position for one repetition (Figure 17-3).

Group 2

Bridging (1 x 15): Supine, knees at 90 degrees, feet on the floor, arms at the sides and hands on ASIS. Maintain neutral and raise the hips until they are in line with the knees. Hold for 3 seconds and return to the floor. Neutral should be maintained through the entire set (Figure 17-4).

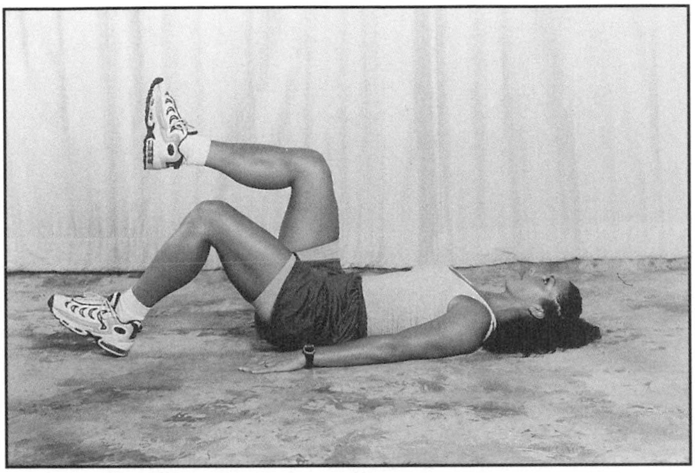

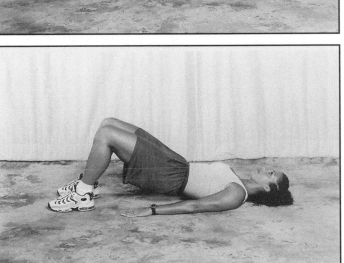

Figure 17-3. Mid-point of one dead bug repetition.

Figure 17-4. Bridge position.

Bridging with leg extension (1 x 10): Supine, knees at 90 degrees, feet on floor, arms at the side and hands on ASIS. Maintain neutral and raise the hips until they are in line with the knees. While holding this position, extend one knee and hold for 2 seconds. Return the leg to the starting position before lowering the pelvis. Repeat the bridge and leg extension on the opposite leg for one repetition (Figure 17-5).

Group 3

Alternating arm and leg (1 x 10): Quadruped position (hands under the shoulders and knees under the hips), maintain neutral, flex the shoulder and extend the contralateral leg simultaneously. Return and perform on opposing limbs for one repetition (Figure 17-6).

Super-person (1 x 10): Prone, pillow under the hips and arms straight out in front. Raise the arms and head off the floor. Hold for 3 seconds and return to the starting position (Figure 17-7).

Figure 17-5. Bridge position with leg extension.

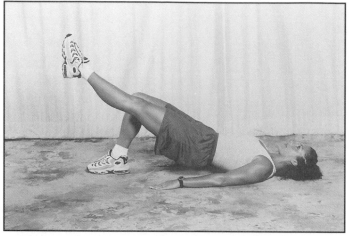

Figure 17-6. Alternating arm and leg in quadruped position.

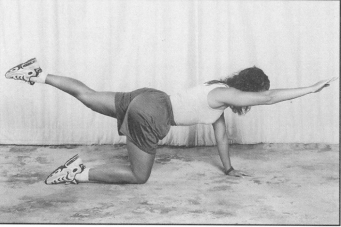

Figure 17-7. Super-person position.

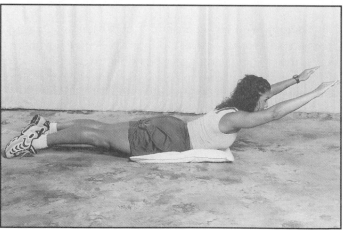

Group 4

Whole body lift, bent elbows (x 2): Prone, maintain neutral, elbows under the shoulders, feet shoulder width apart and raise the body. Only elbows, lower arms, and toes should be in

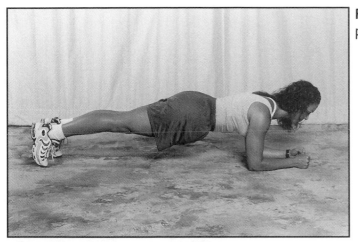

Figure 17-8. Whole body lift position.

contact with the floor. Hold for 30 seconds for one set. Do not allow the shoulders or hips to sag (Figure 17-8).

Whole body lift (x 2): Prone, maintain neutral, hands under the shoulders (push-up position), feet shoulder width apart and raise the body. Only hands and toes should be in contact with the floor. Hold for 30 seconds for one set. Do not allow shoulders or hips to sag.

HIP ROUTINE AND DESCRIPTION

Perform one exercise from each group for a workout routine. Increase repetitions in a set as the workout becomes easy.

Group 1

Bent leg side lift (1 x 20): Quadruped (hands under shoulders and knees under hips), maintain neutral position and raise the flexed knee to side. Maintain stable torso, hip, and knee flexion, then hold for 2 seconds. Continue on the same side until the set is complete. Perform the set on the opposite side (Figure 17-9).

Straight side leg lift (1 x 15): Quadruped (hands under shoulders and knees under hips), maintain neutral position and raise the straight leg to the side. Maintain stable torso and hip flexion, and knee extension, then hold for 2 seconds. Continue on the same side until the set is complete. Perform the set on the opposite side (Figure 17-10).

Repeated side kick (1 x 10): Quadruped (hands under shoulders and knees under hips), maintain neutral position and raise the flexed knee to the side. Hold this position and extend and flex the knee for the entire set of repetitions. Maintain a stable torso and continue until the set is complete. Perform the set on the opposite side (refer to figures 17-9 and 17-10 for sequence).

Figure 17-9. High point of bent leg side lift.

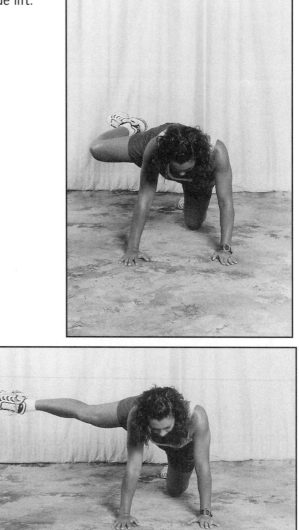

Figure 17-10. High point of straight side leg lift.

Group 2

Straight leg hip extension (1 x 20): Quadruped (hands under shoulders and knees under hips), maintain neutral position and raise the straight leg posteriorly in line with the hips. Hold for 2 seconds. Maintain a stable torso while the extended leg is repeatedly raised. Continue on the same side until the set is complete. Perform set on the opposite side.

Repeated back kick (1 x 30): Quadruped (hands under shoulders and knees under hips), maintain neutral position and raise the straight leg posteriorly in line with the hips. Bring back to start (flexed knee) and repeat extension. Continue on the same side until the set is complete. Perform set on the opposite side.

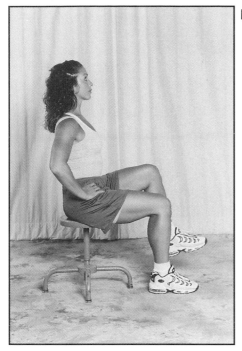

Figure 17-11. High point of seated hip lift.

Group 3

Seated hip lift (1 x 20): Seated, hands on the ASIS, maintain neutral position and raise (flex hip) the foot 4 inches to 6 inches off of floor and hold for 2 seconds. Continue on the same side until the set is complete. Perform the set on the opposite side (Figure 17-11).

Hip circle (1 x 10): Quadruped (hands under shoulders and knees under hips) maintain neutral position. Raise the straight leg posteriorly in line with the hips, swing to the bent leg side position (flexing knee as it moves to the side), and return to quadruped position. One repetition should take a count of three.

LADDER ROUTINE

Secure the ends of "quick foot" or "speed" ladder. Make sure the surface is level and free of debris or obstacles. Appropriate footwear should be emphasized to decrease incidence of abrasions. Drills are meant to increase foot speed, so maintain good form while moving as quickly as possible. Keep the eyes and hips in the direction of movement and perform all drills once up and back on the ladder. Perform drills in sequence without rest. Do not skip or miss any square.

Quick foot (running) forward: Alternate feet, one foot in each square.

Quick feet (running) forward: Lead with one foot up and switch coming back. Both feet land in the same square, but not simultaneously as in a hop.

Lateral shuffle single: Facing one direction (turn to the side), shuffle one foot in each square. Replace the lead foot with the outside foot as it (lead) is moved to the next square. One foot is in a square at a time. Continue to face the same direction and return to start.

Lateral shuffle double: Facing one direction (turn to the side), shuffle two feet in each square. Place the outside foot next to lead before moving the lead to the next square. Feet do not land simultaneously as in a hop, but two feet are in a square at a time. Continue to face the same direction and return to the start.

Hops: Two feet in each square and face forward.

Lateral hops: Facing one direction (turn to the side), hop two feet in each square. Continue to face the same direction and return to start.

Jumping jack hops: Hop in and out of each square with both feet (straddle ladder).

Zig zag double hops: Zig zag, keeping feet together, in the square and out to the side. In square and out to the other side.

Single quick foot: Single leg hops in each square, facing forward (do not alternate). Lead with one leg and switch coming back.

Single zig zag: Zig zag on the single leg, moving in, out, in, out (other side). Switch feet and return to start.

Lateral leading single quick foot: Facing one direction (turn to the side), single leg hop with leading leg in each square. Switch and come back facing the same direction.

Lateral outside single quick foot: Facing one direction (turn to side), single leg hop with outside non-leading leg in each square. Switch and come back facing the same direction.

Zig zag double out: Facing forward, move in a zig zag motion in and out of the squares. Step in (L), in (R/tap, do not step on this foot), out (R), out (L/tap, do not step on this foot), in (L), in (R), and out (L), out (R/tap) to other side.

Zig zag single out: Facing forward, move in a zig zag motion in and out of the squares. Step in (R), in (L), out (R/step), in (L), in(R), out (L/step).

Lateral "W": Facing one direction (turn to the side), step in (lead), in (outside), out (lead), out (outside), and move to the next square. With the left side of the body facing the direction of the movement, step in (lead), in (outside, out (lead), and out (outside). Continue to face the same direction and return to start.

LOWER EXTREMITY PLYOMETRICS DESCRIPTION

Perform all plyometrics on a flat grass surface free of holes or debris. Rest time will vary, but make every effort to wait for full recovery before moving on to the next set. Remember the key to effective and efficient plyometric training is limiting the time spent on the ground.

Warm up: Jog .5 mile or jump rope 5 to 7 minutes, stretch 7 to 10 minutes, walking lunges x 20 yards, ankle hops 2 x 5 yards, straight leg kicks x 20 yards, and skipping x 20 yards.

1. Alternating box bounding: This drill requires two boxes 12 inches to 18 inches in height. Place boxes approximately 6 feet apart (walk through as distances for different athletes will vary) and start about 5 yards in front of and facing the first box. Start with one foot slightly ahead of the other and keep the arms relaxed. Push off the back leg (R), drive the opposite knee toward (L) the chest to gain height and distance. Extend driving knee, land, and bring the back leg (R) forward. Push this leg (R) into the ground and drive the other knee (L), landing on the box. Drive the other (R) forward, landing on the ground. Bound on the ground (L) and drive the back leg forward (R) landing on the box. This sequence completes one repetition. Perform five to 10 repetitions (Figures 17-12a, 17-12b, 17-12c).

2. Alternating leg bounding: Start with one foot slightly ahead of the other and keep the arms relaxed. Push off the back leg (R), drive the opposite knee toward (L) the chest to gain height and distance. Extend the driving knee, land and bring the back leg (R) forward. Extend the driving knee, land, and bring the back leg (L) forward. Perform three to five sets of eight to 12 repetitions. Monitor yardage and strive to increase distance as strength increases.

3. Alternating scissor jumps: Begin in forward lunge position, jump as high and straight as possible using the arms in an upward swing motion. While in the air, switch legs quickly and land in the lunge position with the opposite leg forward for one repetition. Perform two to four sets of eight to 10 repetitions (refer to the lunge in figure A-8).

4. Angled incline hops: To ensure the slope is not too steep, stand in the middle (facing peak) with the feet together and the knees flexed. If balance and comfort can be maintained, then the slope is adequate. Begin at the bottom of a slightly angled slope. Turn 90 degrees in one direction. Keep the feet together, and the knees and hips flexed. Use the arms in an upward swing. Hop quickly and in control up the slope. Walk down the slope and turn 90 degrees in the other direction. Perform two sets of eight to 10 repetitions on each side.

5. Ankle hops: Movement occurs only at the ankles. Hips and knees are extended (body is in an upright position). Keep a large portion of body weight on the balls of the feet and propel forward using small, quick hops. This drill is also used as part of the warm-up routine. Perform one to two sets at 5 yards.

6. Box jumps: This drill requires one box 12 inches to 18 inches in height. Begin by standing close to and in behind box. Keep the feet together, hips and knee slightly flexed. Jump on and off the box quickly. Perform one to three sets of 30 to 60 repetitions.

7. Depth jump: This drill requires one box 12 inches to 18 inches in height. Begin by standing on the box. Step off (do not jump) and land with both feet together and knees flexed. Immediately (this cannot be stressed enough) jump as high as possible. Return to the top of the box. Perform one to three sets of five to 10 repetitions.

8. Double leg bound: Begin with the feet together, hips and knees flexed. Shoulders should be slightly forward. Explode and jump as high and as far as possible. Immediately upon landing, explode and jump again. Perform two to four sets of eight to 12 repetitions. Monitor yardage and strive to increase distance as strength increases.

9. Double leg bound into 20-yard sprint: Begin with the feet together, hips and knees flexed. Shoulders should be slightly forward. Explode and jump as high and as far as possible. Immediately upon landing, explode and jump again. Perform three bounds; upon landing on the third, transfer into a full sprint for 20 yards (one repetition). Perform three to six sets of four repetitions.

10. Double leg box bound: This drill requires two boxes 12 inches to 18 inches in height. Place boxes 3 to 6 feet apart (depending on size of the athlete). Start two steps behind the first box. Shoulders are slightly forward, hips and knees flexed. Use arms in an upward swing motion during propulsion. Explode and jump upward onto the first box. Upon landing, explode and jump upward, landing on the ground. Explode and jump upward onto the sec-

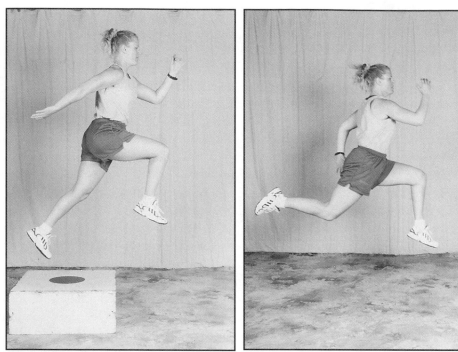

Figure 17-12a. Alternate leg bound from box to ground.

Figure 17-12b. Alternate leg bound on ground.

ond box. Finish the repetition by jumping upward and landing on the ground. Perform two to four sets of three to five repetitions.

11. Double leg speed hops: Stand with flexed knees, chest up, and eyes forward. Shoulders are slightly forward with elbows flexed to 90 degrees. Jump up as high as possible, flex the knees completely forward to bring the feet under hips. Bring the knees high and forward with each hop. Distance is not a factor here. Perform two to five sets of 10 to 20 repetitions.

12. Ice skaters: Mark off a distance (using tape or cones) of three. Begin standing in the middle with hips and knees flexed. Remain close to the ground during the drill. Push off to land on a single leg just outside marker. From this position, push off to land on a single leg just outside other (3 feet away) marker for one repetition. Perform two to four sets of eight to 10 repetitions (Figure 17-13).

13. Incline hops: To ensure the slope is not too steep, stand in the middle (facing peak) with the feet together and knees flexed. If balance and comfort can be maintained, then the slope is adequate. Begin at the bottom of a slightly angled slope. Keep feet together, knees and hips flexed. Use the arms in an upward swing. Hop up the slope quickly and in control. Walk down the slope. Perform two sets of eight to 10 repetitions.

14. Jump rope routine: Perform each exercise as a 30-second sprint. Rest 30 seconds between exercises. With single leg exercises, keep the non-moving thigh parallel to the floor.

- Two feet jumping
- Two feet side to side over line
- Two feet front and back over line
- One foot jumping, change (no rest between single leg exercises)

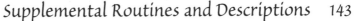

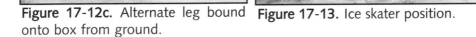

Figure 17-12c. Alternate leg bound onto box from ground.   **Figure 17-13.** Ice skater position.

- One foot side to side over line, change (no rest between single leg exercises)
- One foot front and back over line, change (no rest between single leg exercises)
- Two feet jumping four squares (change direction)
- Two feet jump three regular spins and one double spin, continue
- Two feet jump consecutive double spins

15. Lateral box jumps: This drill requires one box 6 inches to 12 inches in height. Standing (approximately 6 inches) to one side of the box, turn 90 degrees so the feet are parallel with the box. Continue facing one direction until the set is complete. Jump on and off the box quickly. Recover and turn to face the other direction, jump on and off the box quickly. Perform one to three sets (each way) for 10 to 20 repetitions.

16. Lateral box jumps across the box: This drill requires one box 12 inches to 18 inches in height. Standing (approximately 6 inches) to one side of the box, turn 90 degrees so the feet are parallel with the box. Jump onto the box and off, landing on the opposite side for one repetition. Continue back and forth for the entire set. Perform one to three sets of five to 10 repetitions (Figures 17-14a, 14b, and 14c).

17. Lateral cone hops: This drill requires one cone 12 inches to 24 inches in height. Standing to one side of the cone, jump over and back for one repetition. Perform two to four sets of 10 to 20 repetitions.

18. Power skipping: Skip as high and as far as possible. Drive the front leg high. Push and extend the propelling leg. Swing the opposite arm with the driving leg. One power skip is one repetition. Perform one to three sets of eight to 12 repetitions (Figure 17-15).

19. Repeated cone/hurdle hops: This drill requires either four cones or four hurdles. Keep

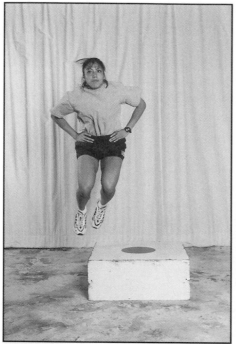

Figure 17-14a. Lateral box jump from ground onto box.

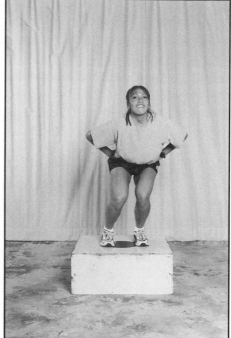

Figure 17-14b. Box land and take-off position.

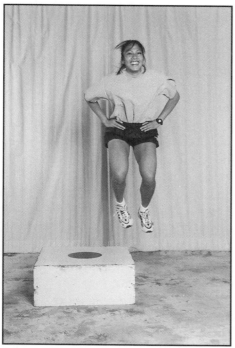

Figure 17-14c. Continued lateral box jump from box to ground.

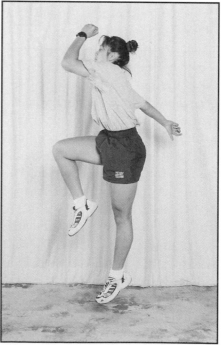

Figure 17-15. High point of power skip.

the feet together, hips and knees flexed. Use the arms in an upward swing motion during propulsion. Jump up and over each implement, walk back to the start for one repetition. Do not take extra steps between implements; movement should be continuous. Perform four to six sets of four repetitions.

20. Repeated cone/hurdle hops into 20-yard sprint: This drill requires either four cones or four hurdles. Keep the feet together, hips and knees flexed. Use the arms in an upward swing motion during propulsion. Jump up and over each implement, then full sprint for 20 yards. Do not take extra steps between implements; movement should be continuous. Perform two to four sets of four repetitions.

21. Repeated lateral cone hops: This drill requires four cones. Standing to one side of the cone, keep the feet together, hips and knees flexed. Use the arms in an upward swing motion during propulsion. Jump up and over each cone, jump back over cones, facing the same direction for one repetition. Do not take extra steps between cones; movement should be continuous. Perform two to four sets of four repetitions.

22. Repeated single lateral cone hops with leading leg: This drill requires four relatively small cones. Use the arms in an upward swing motion during propulsion. Jump up and over each cone with the lead leg, switch feet and jump back over the cones, facing the same direction for one repetition. Do not take extra steps between implements; movement should be continuous. Perform two to four sets of four repetitions.

23. Repeated single lateral cone hops with outside leg: This drill requires four relatively small cones. Use the arms in an upward swing motion during propulsion. Jump up and over each cone with the outside leg, switch feet, and jump back over cones, facing the same direction for one repetition. Do not take extra steps between implements; movement should be continuous. Perform two to four sets of four repetitions.

24. Single lateral cone hops: This drill requires one relatively small cone. Standing to one side of the cone, jump over and back with a single leg for one repetition. Perform two to four sets of eight to 12 repetitions.

25. Single leg bound: Start with a running start (10 yards) and bound with a single leg. One leg should be held in a stationary flexed position throughout the bounding drill. Use a double arm swing and jump as high and far as possible. Perform three to five sets of eight to 12 repetitions. Monitor yardage and strive to increase distance as strength increases.

26. Single leg bound into 20-yard sprint: Start with a running start (10 yards) and bound with a single leg. One leg should be held in a stationary flexed position throughout the bounding drill. Use a double arm swing and jump as high and far as possible. Complete four bounds, then full sprint for 20 yards for one repetition. Perform two to four sets of three repetitions on each leg.

27. Single leg box jumps: This drill requires one box 6 inches to 12 inches in height. Begin by standing close to and behind the box. Keep one leg stationary, hips and knees slightly flexed. Jump on and off the box quickly with a single leg, switch feet. Perform one to three sets of 10 to 20 repetitions.

28. Single leg lateral box jumps: This drill requires one box 6 inches in height. Standing (approximately 6 inches) to one side of the box, turn 90 degrees so the feet are parallel with the box. Continue facing one direction until the set is complete. Keep one leg stationary, hips and knees slightly flexed. Jump on and off the box quickly with a single leg until set is complete. Turn to face the other direction, jump on and off the box quickly. Perform one to three sets (each way) for 10 to 20 repetitions.

29. Single leg speed hops: Stand with flexed knees. Shoulders are slightly forward with elbows flexed to 90 degrees. Jump up as high as possible; keep one leg stationary. Use a double arm; swing and flex the knee completely forward to bring the foot under the hips. Bring the knee high and forward with each hop. Distance is not a factor here. Perform two to five sets of five to 15 repetitions.

30. Skipping: Quick skipping, steps are short and feet are kept close to the ground and land simultaneously. Emphasis is on driving into the ground. Perform two sets of 10 yards.

31. Split jumps: Begin in a forward lunge position; jump as high and straight as possible using the arms in an upward swing motion. When landing, retain the lunge position and flex the knees to absorb shock. Continue on the same side until the set is complete, then switch legs. Perform two to four sets of 10 to 15 repetitions (Refer to lunge in Figure A-8).

32. Standing long jump: Stand with flexed knees. Shoulders are slightly forward with elbows flexed to 90 degrees. Flex knees and hips further and jump outward as far as possible for one repetition. Regain stance and jump again. Height is not a factor, but distance is. Perform one to three sets of five to eight repetitions. Monitor distance as strength increases.

33. Straight leg kicks: Stand with the hands on the hips and the knees extended in an upright position. Stay on the balls of the feet and maintain extended knees. Alternate kicking legs out in front of the body. Feet should not rise more than 12 inches off of the ground. This drill is only used as part of the warm-up routine. Perform one to two sets of 20 yards.

MEDICINE BALL ROUTINE AND DESCRIPTION

A medicine ball routine should be performed in a wide-open area free of equipment or obstacles. The size, strength, and experience level of the athlete should be instrumental when choosing a medicine ball weight. Beginners and those performing one arm movements should use a 2-to-6 pound ball. More advanced and stronger athletes may use six to 15 pounds. The catch phase is similar to that of the landing in the lower extremity plyometrics. Emphasis should be on quickness and technique. Very little time should be spent during the catch phase.

Chest pass: Stand, knees slightly flexed, and hold the ball with both hands at chest level. Hyperextend the back slightly, keep the elbows out and pass the ball to a partner. Elbows should now be fully extended, palms facing away from the body, and wrists flexed. Your partner will then pass the ball back to you. Catch pass with flexed elbows for one repetition. Increase distance between partners to increase difficulty. Perform two sets of 10 repetitions.

Chest pass with lunge: Kneel (with pad) and hold ball with both hands at chest level. Hyperextend back slightly, keep elbows out, pass ball to partner and fall forward. Absorb body weight with flexed elbows in push-up position. Perform one to two sets of 10 to 15 repetitions.

Chest pass with step: Stand, knees slightly flexed, and hold the ball with both hands at chest level. Hyperextend the back slightly, keep the elbows out, pass the ball to a partner and step out with one leg. Pass and step are executed simultaneously. Elbows should now be fully extended, palms facing away from the body, and wrists flexed. Your partner will pass the ball back to you. Catch pass with flexed elbows for one repetition. Change legs between repetitions. Increase distance between partners to increase difficulty. Perform one to two sets of 10 to 20 repetitions.

Kneeling chest pass: Kneel (with a pad) and hold the ball with both hands at chest level. Hyperextend the back slightly, keep the elbows out, pass the ball to a partner. Elbows should now be fully extended, palms facing away from the body, and wrists flexed. Your partner will pass the ball back to you. Catch pass with flexed elbows for one repetition. Increase distance between partners to increase difficulty. Perform one to two sets of 10 to 20 repetitions.

Kneeling overhead pass: Kneel (with a pad) and hold the ball with both hands at chest level. Bring the ball behind the head and pass it to a partner. Elbows should now be fully extended, palms facing away from the body, and wrists flexed. Your partner will pass the ball back to you. Catch pass at chest level with flexed elbows for one repetition. Increase distance between partners to increase difficulty. Perform one to two sets of 10 to 15 repetitions.

One arm pass: Stand, knees slightly flexed, hold ball with both hands. Twist (keep hips straight) to one side and push/pass with that side's hand. Your partner will pass the ball back to you. Catch pass at chest level (facing a partner) with flexed elbows for one repetition. Twist to the other side and push/pass with that side's hand. Increase distance between partners to increase difficulty. Perform one to two sets of 20 to 30 repetitions.

One arm toss: Stand, knees slightly flexed, hold the ball with one hand. Abduct and externally rotate the shoulder to 90 degrees. From this position, externally rotate slightly more (with some torso twist) and toss to a partner. Your partner will pass the ball back to you. Catch pass at chest level with flexed elbows for one repetition. Switch hands and perform same movement. Increase distance between partners to increase difficulty. Perform two to four sets of 20 to 30 repetitions.

Overhead pass: Stand, knees slightly flexed, and hold the ball with both hands at chest level. Bring the ball behind the head and pass it to a partner. Elbows should now be fully extended, palms facing away from the body and wrists flexed. Your partner will pass the ball back to you. Catch pass at chest level with flexed elbows for one repetition. Increase distance between partners to increase difficulty. Perform one to two sets of 10 to 15 repetitions.

Overhead pass with lunge: Kneel (with pad) and hold the ball with both hands at chest level. Bring the ball behind the head and pass the ball to a partner. Keep the elbows out, pass the ball to a partner and fall forward. Absorb body weight with flexed elbows in push-up position. Your partner will then pass the ball back to you. Catch pass at chest level with flexed elbows for one repetition. Increase distance between partners to increase difficulty. Perform one to two sets of 10 to 15 repetitions.

Overhead pass with step: Stand, knees slightly flexed, and hold the ball with both hands at chest level. Bring the ball behind the head, pass it to a partner and step out with one leg. Pass and step are executed simultaneously. Elbows should now be fully extended, palms facing away from the body, and wrists flexed. Your partner will then pass the ball back to you. Catch pass at chest level with flexed elbows for one repetition. Increase distance between partners to increase difficulty. Perform one to two sets of 10 to 15 repetitions.

Overhead toss: Stand with the back facing the target. Squat and allow the ball to lower between the legs. Jump upward as high as possible while tossing the ball behind the head as far as possible. Perform one to two sets of five to 15 repetitions.

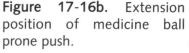
Figure 17-16a. Start and finish positions of medicine ball prone push.

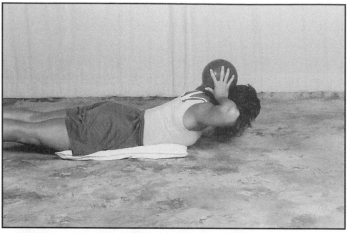

Figure 17-16b. Extension position of medicine ball prone push.

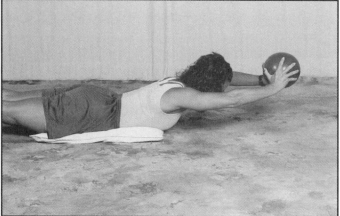

Prone push: Lie prone with a pillow under the hips. Begin with a (light) ball behind the head. Extend the back so the chest is off the ground. Push the ball forward so the elbows are fully extended. Maintain back extension during the entire set. Perform one to two sets of five to 10 repetitions (Figures 17-16a, 17-16b).

Push-up: In the push-up position, place one hand on the ball and one hand on the ground (or both hands on one ball). Maintain a stable torso and lower the chest to the ground (or ball). Switch sides after completion of a set. Perform two to three sets of two to 15 repetitions (Figure 17-17).

Squat push: Stand facing the target and hold the ball with both hands at chest level. Squat jump and during ascension, push the ball up and forward with force. Perform one to three sets of eight to 12 repetitions.

Supine drops: Lying supine, a partner stands over and above the head. The partner drops the ball, catch it with flexed elbows. Immediately push the ball in the air. Elbows should now be fully extended, palms facing away from the body, and wrists flexed. Perform two to four sets of 10 to 15 repetitions (Figures 17-18a and 18b).

Walk over: Place the ball outside of the hands and assume the push-up position. Place the inside hand on the ball and hold. Place the outside hand on the ball and hold (both hands

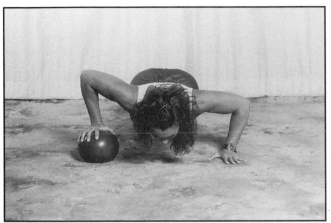

Figure 17-17. Descent position of medicine ball push up.

should be on the ball). Now move inside and hand off, then outside and hand off. Walk over to the other side for one repetition. Perform one to two sets of four to eight repetitions.

RICE ROUTINE

This routine is performed sitting or kneeling in front of a large 15 to 25 gallon bucket of rice. Perform exercises in sequence without rest.

Finger jabs: With extended fingers, palms facing each other, jab hard and quickly in and out of the rice. The rice should cover the wrists. Hands should exit the rice after each repetition. Perform two sets of 20 repetitions.

Rice grab: With extended fingers, pronated forearms, quickly squeeze (grab) the rice. Rice should cover the wrists. Hands stay submerged during entire set. Perform three sets of 30 repetitions.

Kneading in: Grab and turn from pronation to supination. The rice should cover the wrists. Hands should exit the rice after each repetition. Perform two sets of 30 repetitions.

Kneading out: Grab and turn from supination to pronation. The rice should cover the wrists. Hands should exit the rice after each repetition. Perform two sets of 30 repetitions.

ROTATOR CUFF WARM-UP ROUTINE

This routine is performed holding 2.5-to-5ive pound dumbbells. Do not exceed 5 pounds. This will ensure limited involvement of the deltoid muscles. Perform exercises in sequence without rest. This warm-up may also be performed using secured elastic tubing.

Front raise: Stand, feet shoulder width apart and knees slightly flexed. Hold the weight with the palms facing each other, flex shoulders fully (over head) and control descent. Perform one set of 12 repetitions.

Reverse lateral raise: Stand, feet shoulder width apart and knees slightly flexed. Grip the weight with the palms facing each other, abduct the shoulders to 90 degrees, externally rotate the shoulders and continue abduction (with palms facing up) to 180 degrees. Weight should be overhead and palms facing each other. Internally rotate at 90 degrees during descent (palms facing down) and finish with palms facing each other. Perform one set of 12 repetitions in each direction.

Empty soda can: Stand, feet shoulder width apart and knees slightly flexed. Abduct the shoulders to 90 degrees, horizontally adduct 45 degrees, then internally rotate so the thumbs are pointing to the floor (elbows are slightly flexed). Lower and raise the weight in a controlled manner without raising it beyond parallel with the floor. Perform one set of 12 repetitions.

External rotation: Stand, feet shoulder width apart and knees slightly flexed. Abduct shoulders to 90 degrees and flex the elbows to 90 degrees. Maintain this position and externally rotate the shoulders. Return to starting position, keeping the arms parallel with the floor. Perform one set of 12 repetitions.

Internal/external rotation: Side lie with a flexed (90 degrees) elbow slightly off the bench. Internally rotate the shoulder fully. Maintain this position and switch the dumbbell into the outside hand. Externally rotate the shoulder fully. Continue with the same movement until the set is complete. Side lie on the other side and repeat internal/external rotation. Perform one set of 12 repetitions in each direction.

ISOMETRIC EXERCISES

Flexed arm hang: Body is positioned and holds at completion of a pull-up. This allows the athlete to experience what the finish feels like, especially if he/she is unable to complete one solo.

Single leg stand: Stationary standing with one leg (extended knee) initiates the muscles that support the ankle. This could possibly decrease the severity of an ankle sprain.

Single leg stand with heel raise: Heel is raised off the floor (extended knee) and held in a stationary position. This not only strengthens the posterior compartment at its weakest point in the range of motion, but also provides a little advanced balance training.

Wall sit: Torso is positioned against a wall with the hips and knees flexed to 90 degrees. This may also benefit the lifter who has difficulty at the bottom of the power squat, or for the athlete who has to hold a position similar to this, such as a speed skater, defensive volleyball or basketball player, or offensive lineman.

Whole body lift: Described in the back stabilization program, this increases torso stability, along with shoulder and hip stability. Very applicable to anyone. Even the recreational sports person or office worker benefits from a good stable torso.

ISOTONIC EXERCISES

Examples of "Machine" Whole Body Circuits

Example #1
1. Leg press

Example #2
1. Pec deck/fly

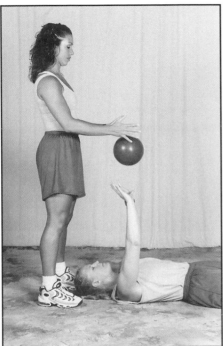

Figure 17-18a. Medicine ball dropping from a standing partner in supine drop.

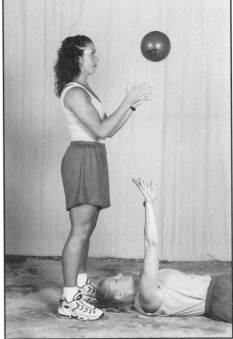

Figure 17-18b. Medicine ball accelerating from a lying partner in supine drop.

2. Seated bench press
3. Cable upright row
4. Lat pulldown
5. Dips
6. Cable bicep curl
7. Abdominal crunches
8. Pelvic tilts
9. Seated calf raises

2. Seated row
3. Seated military press
4. Leg extension
5. Leg curl
6. Tricep pushdown
7. Cable reverse bicep curl
8. Roman chair leg lifts
9. Standing calf raises

Examples of Free-Weight Isotonic Exercises

Lower body: DB squats, lunges (forward, lateral, cross-over), step-ups, stiff-legged dead lift, hang cleans, calf raises.

Chest: DB bench press, incline press, lying flys, incline flys.

Shoulders: DB military press, front raise, lateral raise, reverse lateral raise, bent-over front raise, bent-over lateral raise, upright row, shrugs.

Back: DB bent-over row, pullover, one arm row.

Biceps: DB curl, hammer curl, seated curl, incline curl.

Triceps: DB tricep extension, lying tricep extension, kick back.

For a complete list of exercises, please refer to the weightlifting descriptions in the Appendix.

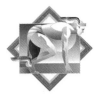

Chapter Eighteen

Sport-Specific Programs

The following pages contain specific programs for various sports. The sports are alphabetized and with the phases in appropriate sequence. Please refer to Chapter Five for assistance in determining percentages for sets and repetitions and how many weeks each phase should run. Please also refer to Chapter Seventeen for the supplemental routines and the Appendix for the weightlifting descriptions. The numbers after the plyometric and medicine ball routines correspond to the appropriate drills found in Chapter Seventeen.

For all of the sport-specific strength training programs, the following key applies:

SS = super-set
TS = tri-set

A super-set involves two exercises. In these example programs, super-set the exercise with the "SS" and the exercise directly preceding it. The participant performs one set of the first exercise and immediately follows with a set of the second exercise. It is after the two sets that the rest period takes place. This alternating pattern is repeated until the sets have been completed.

A tri-set involves three exercises. In these example programs, tri-set the exercise with the "TS" and the exercises directly preceding and following it.

The participant performs one set of the first exercise, immediately follows with a set of the second exercise and third exercise. It is after the three sets that the rest period takes place. This pattern is repeated until the sets have been completed.

BASEBALL/SOFTBALL (INFIELDERS)

Introduction Phase

Day 1
Rotator Cuff Warm-up	x 2
Push-ups	1 x 10
Incline Push-ups	1 x 10
Bench Press	3 x 12
Incline Press	3 x 12
DB Incline Flys	3 x 15
DB Standing Military	3 x 10
DB Bent-over Front Raises	3 x 10
DB Bent-over Lateral Raises	3 x 10 SS
Bench Dips	3 x 20
Tricep Push-down	3 x 15
Rice Routine	
Abdominal #1	

Day 3
Rotator cuff warm-up	x 2
Push-ups	1 x 10
Decline Push-ups	1 x 10
DB Bench Press	3 x 15
DB Lying Flys	3 x 15
DB Incline Press	3 x 12
Upright Rows	3 x 12
DB Front Raises	3 x 15
DB Lateral Raises	3 x 15 SS
Dips	3 x 10
DB Tricep Extension	3 x 12
Rice Routine	
Abdominal #2	

Day 2
Rotator Cuff Warm-up	x 2
Pull-ups	2 x 8
Good Mornings	2 x 15 TS
Torso Twists	2 x 20
High Pulls	3 x 10
Leg Sled	3 x 12
Lateral Lunges	2 x 10
Leg Curls	2 x 10 SS
T-Bar Rows	3 x 12
Lat Pull-downs	3 x 15
DB Incline Curls	3 x 12
Straight Bar Curls	3 x 15
Seated Calves	2 x 25
Hip Routine	
Back Stabilization	

Day 4
Rotator Cuff Warm-up	x 2
Pull-ups	2 x 8
DB Stiff Leg Dead Lift	2 x 15 TS
Torso Twists	2 x 20
Hang Cleans	3 x 10
Squat	3 x 10
Walking Lunges	2 x 10
Leg Curls	2 x 15 SS
Pull-overs	3 x 15
Seated Rows	3 x 15
DB Incline Hammer Curl	3 x 10
E-Z Bar Curl	3 x 12
Standing Calves, Single	2 x 25
Hip Routine	
Back Stabilization	

Strength Phase

Day 1	
Rotator Cuff Warm-up	x 2
Push-ups	1 x 15
Decline Push-ups	1 x 15
Bench Press	1 x 10, 2 x 8
DB Incline Flys	2 x 12
Military Press	3 x 10
DB Reverse Lateral Raises	2 x 12
DB Shrugs	2 x 12 SS
Bench Dips	3 x 15
Rice Routine	
Abdominal #1	
Ladder	1 set

Day 3	
Rotator Cuff Warm-up	x 2
Push-ups	2 x 10
Incline Push-ups	2 x 15 SS
DB Incline Press	3 x 10
DB Lying Flys	2 x 12
DB Standing Military	2 x 10
DB Bent-over Front Raises	3 x 10
DB Upright Rows	3 x 10 SS
DB Tricep Extension	3 x 10
Rice Routine	
Abdominal #2	
Ladder	1 set

Day 2	
Rotator Cuff Warm-up	x 2
Pull-ups	2 x 10
Good Mornings	2 x 15 TS
Torso Twists	2 x 20 TS
Power Cleans	3 x 8
Leg Sled	3 x 10
Step-ups	2 x 10
Pull-overs	3 x 8
Seated Rows	2 x 10
DB Hammer Curls	3 x 12
Seated Calves	2 x 25
Hip Routine	
Back Stabilization	

Day 4	
Rotator Cuff Warm-up	x 2
Pull-ups	2 x 10
Twisting Back Extension	2 x 10 TS
Torso Twists	2 x 20 TS
Hang Cleans	2 x 8
Squat	3 x 8
DB One Arm Rows	3 x 10
Straight Bar Pull-downs	3 x 10 SS
Leg Extensions	2 x 10
Leg Curls	2 x 10 SS
Single Standing Calves	2 x 30
Hip Routine	
Back Stabilization	

Power Phase

Day 1	
Rotator Cuff Warm-up	x 2
Decline Push-ups	2 x 15
DB Lying Flys	2 x 15 SS
DB Bench Press	1 x 8, 2 x 6
DB Standing Military	3 x 8
DB Bent-over Front Raises	3 x 10

Day 3	
Rotator Cuff Warm-up	x 2
Decline Push-ups	2 x 15
DB Incline Flys	2 x 15 SS
Wide Grip Bench Press	3 x 10
DB Pull-overs	3 x 10 SS
DB Upright Rows	3 x 10

DB Bent-over Lateral Raises	3 x 10	Cable Front Raises	3 x 10
Bench Dips	2 x 20	Cable Lateral Raises	3 x 10
DB Tricep Extension	2 x 8	DB Hammer Curls	3 x 10
Rice Routine		Rice Routine	
Ladder	1 Set	Ladder	1 Set
Plyometrics #'s	2, 12, 16, 28	Plyometrics #'s	20, 22, 23, 27

Day 2		Day 4	
Rotator Cuff Warm-up	x 1	Rotator Cuff Warm-up	x 1
Pull-ups	2 x 8	Pull-ups	2 x 8
Good Mornings	2 x 15 TS	Good Mornings	2 x 15TS
Torso Twists	2 x 20	Torso Twists	2 x 20
Power Cleans	1 x 8, 2 x 6	Squat	1 x 8, 2 x 6
Walking Lunges	2 x 10	Lateral Lunges	3 x 10
Squat Jumps	2 x 10 TS	Lateral Cone Hops	2 x 10 SS
Leg Curls	2 x 10	Leg Curls	3 x 10
T-Bar Rows	3 x 8	Seated Rows	3 x 10
Straight Bar Pull-downs	3 x 10	Abdominal #1	
Abdominal #2		Slide Board	2 x 40
Slide Board	2 x 40	Back Stabilization	
Back Stabilization		Med Ball Routine #'s	7, 9, 16
Med Ball Routine #'s	5, 6, 13		

Peak/Transition Phase

Day 1		Day 3	
Rotator Cuff Warm-up	x 2	Rotator Cuff Warm-up	x 2
Med Ball Push-ups	2 x 10 (R/L)	UE Step-ups	2 x 10
Torso Twists	2 x 20 SS	Torso Twists	2 x 20 SS
DB Bench Press	1 x 8, 1 x 6, 1 x 4	Wide Grip Bench Press	3 x 8
DB Lying Flys	3 x 10	DB Incline Press	3 x 8
Med Ball Single Arm Toss	3 x 10 SS	Med Ball Overhead Pass	3 x 10 SS
DB Military Press	2 x 10	DB Upright Row	3 x 8
DB Bent-over Front Raise	2 x 10	DB Front Raise	2 x 10
Rear Deltoid Pull	2 x 10 SS	DB Lateral Raise	2 x 10 SS
Bench Dips	2 x 20	Dips	2 x 10
Straight Bar Curl	2 x 10 SS	DB Hammer Curl	2 x 10
Abdominal #		Med Ball Abdominal	
Plyometrics #'s	1, 3, 10, 11	Plyometrics #'s	12, 25, 29

Day 2		Day 4	
Rotator Cuff Warm-up	x 1	Rotator Cuff Warm-up	x 1

Pull-ups	2 x 10	Pull-ups	2 x 10
Good Mornings	2 x 15 SS	Stiff Leg Dead Lift	2 x 10 SS
Power Cleans	1 x 8, 1 x 6, 1 x 4	Hang Cleans	2 x 8
Squat	1 x 8, 1 x 6, 1 x 4	Leg Sled	1 x 8, 1 x 6, 1 x 4
Ice Skaters	3 x 10 SS	Lateral Box Jumps	3 x 10 SS
Seated Rows	3 x 8	Lat Pull-downs (ALT)	3 x 10
Back Stabilization		Back Stabilization	
Ladder	1 set	Ladder	1 set
Slide Board	1 x 30	Slide Board	1 x 30
Med Ball Routine #'s	2, 7, 9	Med Ball Routine #'s	10, 12

BASEBALL/SOFTBALL (OUTFIELDERS)

Introduction Phase

Day 1

Rotator Cuff Warm-up	x 2
Good Mornings	2 x 15
Torso Twists	2 x 20 SS
DB Hang Cleans	2 x 10
Leg Sled	3 x 15
Step-ups	2 x 12
Leg Curls	2 x 15 SS
Pull-overs	3 x 10
Seated Rows	3 x 15 SS
Seated Calves	2 x 25
Hip Routine	
Back Stabilization	

Day 3

Rotator Cuff Warm-up	x 2
Pull-ups	2 x 10
Torso Twists	2 x 20 SS
High Pulls	3 x 10
Walking Lunges	2 x 10
DB Stiff Leg Dead Lift	2 x 15 TS
Leg Curls	2 x 15
Straight Bar Pull-downs	3 x 15
DB One Arm Rows	3 x 10
Standing Calves, Single	2 x 25
Hip Routine	
Back Stabilization	

Day 2

Rotator Cuff Warm-up	x 2
Push-ups	2 x 10
DB Lying Flys	2 x 15 SS
Bench Press	3 x 12
Military Press	3 x 15
Upright Rows	2 x 15
DB Reverse Lateral Raises	2 x 12 SS
Bench Dips	3 x 15
DB Hammer Curls	3 x 10 SS

Day 4

Rotator Cuff Warm-up	x 2
Decline Push-ups	2 x 10
DB Incline Flys	2 x 15 SS
DB Bench Press	3 x 15
DB Upright Rows	3 x 15
Rear Deltoid Pull	3 x 15
DB Lateral Raises	3 x 15 SS
Dips	2 x 8
DB Tricep Extension	3 x 15

Straight Bar Curls	2 x 10	E-Z Bar Curls	3 x 10 SS
Rice Routine		Rice Routine	
Abdominal #1		Abdominal #2	

Strength Phase

Day 1		Day 3	
Rotator Cuff Warm-up	x 2	Rotator Cuff Warm-up	x 2
Pull-ups	2 x 10	Pull-ups	2 x 10
Back Extension	2 x 10	Twisting Back Extension	2 x 10
Power Cleans	3 x 8	Hang Cleans	3 x 8
Squat	3 x 8	Leg Sled	3 x 8
Lunges	2 x 10	Lateral Lunges	2 x 10
Leg Curls	2 x 10 SS	Leg Curls	2 x 10 SS
Seated Rows	3 x 10	DB Pull-overs	2 x 10
Straight Bar Pull-downs	3 x 10 SS	T-Bar Rows	3 x 10
Seated Calves	2 x 25	Standing Calves, Single	2 x 30
Hip Routine		Hip Routine	
Back Stabilization		Back Stabilization	

Day 2		Day 4	
Rotator Cuff Warm-up	x 2	Rotator Cuff Warm-up	x 2
Decline Push-ups	1 x 15	Push-ups	2 x 15
Torso Twists	1 x 20	Torso Twists	2 x 20 SS
DB Bench Press	3 x 8	DB Incline Press	3 x 8
DB Lying Flys	3 x 10	DB Incline Flys	3 x 10
Military Press	3 x 10	DB Upright Rows	2 x 10
Cable Front Raises	2 x 10	DB Shrugs	2 x 10 SS
Cable Lateral Raises	2 x 10	DB Bent-over Lateral Raises	3 x 10
Bench Dips	2 x 15	Straight Bar Curl	2 x 10
DB Tricep Extension	3 x 10	DB Hammer Curl	3 x 10
Rice Routine		Rice Routine	
Abdominal #1		Abdominal #2	

Power Phase

Day 1		Day 3	
Rotator Cuff Warm-up	x 2	Rotator Cuff Warm-up	x 2
Pull-ups	2 x 10	Pull-ups	2 x 10
Twisting Back Extension	2 x 20	Torso Twists	2 x 20
DB Stiff Leg Dead Lift	2 x 15 SS	Hang Cleans	3 x 5
Power Cleans	1 x 8, 2 x 6	DB Squat Jumps	2 x 8 SS

Lateral Lunges	3 x 10	Walking Lunges	2 x 10
Seated Rows	3 x 8	DB Pull-overs	3 x 8
Straight Bar Pull-downs	3 x 10	T-Bar Rows	3 x 8
Straight Bar Curls	3 x 10	DB Incline Hammer Curls	3 x 10
Seated Calves	2 x 25	Single Standing Calves	2 x 30
Med Ball Routine #'s	5, 6, 8	Med Ball Routine #'s	10, 14, 16

Day 2		Day 4	
Rotator Cuff Warm-up	x 2	Rotator Cuff Warm-up	x 2
Med Ball Push-ups	2 x 10	Decline Push-ups	2 x 15
Dips	2 x 10	Med Ball Chest Pass	2 x 10 SS
DB Lying Flys (Light)	2 x 15	Good Mornings	2 x 15
DB Bench Press	1 x 8, 2 x 6	DB Incline Press	1 x 8, 2 x 6
Rear Military Press	3 x 8	DB Standing Military Press	3 x 8
Upright Rows	3 x 8	DB Bent-over Front Raises	3 x 10
DB Bent-over Lateral Raises	3 x 10	DB Reverse Lateral Raises	3 x 10 SS
Tricep Push-down	3 x 10	DB Lying Tricep Extension	3 x 10
Med Ball Abdominal		Abdominal #2	
Back Stabilization		Back Stabilization	
Plyometrics #'s	2, 8, 9, 12	Plyometrics #'s	16, 18, 20, 26

Peak/Transition Phase

Day 1		Day 3	
Rotator Cuff Warm-up	x 2	Rotator Cuff Warm-up	x 2
Pull-ups	2 x 5	Pull-ups	2 x 5
Torso Twists	2 x 10	Torso Twists	2 x 10
Good Mornings	2 x 20 TS	Good Mornings	2 x 20 TS
Twisting Back Extension	2 x 20	Twisting Back Extension	2 x 20
Power Cleans	1 x 8, 1 x 6, 2 x 3	Hang Cleans	3 x 5
Lateral Box Jumps	4 x 10 SS	Leg Sled	1 x 8, 1 x 6, 2 x 3
Walking Lunges	2 x 10	Ice Skaters	4 x 20 SS
Leg Curls	2 x 10 SS	DB One Arm Rows	3 x 8
Seated Rows	3 x 8	Pull-overs	3 x 8
Back Stabilization		Back Stabilization	
Med Ball Routine #'s	5, 7, 9	Med Ball Routine #'s	10, 16

Day 2		Day 4	
Rotator Cuff Warm-up	x 2	Rotator Cuff Warm-up	x 2
Decline Push-ups	2 x 15	Push-ups	2 x 15

UE Step-ups	2 x 10 SS	Med Ball Over-head Pass	2 x 10 SS
Dips	2 x 10	Dips	2 x 10
DB Incline Flys	2 x 15 SS	DB Lying Flys	2 x 15 SS
Wide Grip Bench Press	2 x 10	DB Incline Press	1 x 8, 1 x 6, 2 x 3
DB Bench Press	1 x 8, 1 x 6, 2 x 3	DB Military Press	3 x 8
DB Upright Rows	3 x 8	DB Front Raises	3 x 8
DB Shrugs	3 x 8 SS	DB Lateral Raises	3 x 8 SS
DB Hammer Curls	3 x 10	DB Curls	3 x 10
Abdominal #1		Med Ball Abdominal	
Plyometrics #'s	1, 9, 11	Plyometrics #'s	20, 27, 29

BASEBALL/SOFTBALL (PITCHERS)

Introduction Phase

Day 1		Day 3	
Rotator Cuff Warm-up	x 2	Rotator Cuff Warm-up	x 2
Push-ups	2 x 10	Decline Push-ups	2 x 10
DB Incline Press	3 x 10	DB Bench Press	3 x 15
DB Incline Flys	3 x 15	DB Lying Flys	3 x 15
Military Press	3 x 12	DB Standing Military	3 x 10
Upright Rows	3 x 15	DB Reverse Lateral Raises	3 x 12
DB Bent-over Front Raises	3 x 12	DB Bent-over Lateral Raises	3 x 12 SS
DB Incline Hammer Curls	3 x 10	Straight Bar Curls	3 x 15
Bench Dips	3 x 15	DB Hammer Curls	3 x 10
DB Tricep Extension	3 x 10	Dips	3 x 8
Rice Routine	x 2	Rice Routine	x 2
Abdominal #1		Abdominal #2	

Day 2		Day 4	
Rotator Cuff Warm-up	x 2	Rotator Cuff Warm-up	x 2
Pull-ups	2 x 5	Pull-ups	2 x 5
Good Morning	2 x 15 TS	DB Stiff Leg Dead Lift	2 x 15 TS
Torso Twists	2 x 15	Twisting Back Extension	2 x 12
High Pulls	3 x 10	Power Squat	3 x 12
Single Leg Sled	3 x 15	Push Press	3 x 8
Walking Lunges	3 x 10	Step-ups	3 x 10
Leg Curls	3 x 15 SS	Single Leg Curls	3 x 10 SS
Seated Row	3 x 15	DB One Arm Rows	3 x 15

Pull-overs	3 x 12 SS	Lat Pull-down	3 x 12
Standing Calves, Single	2 x 25	Seated Calves	3 x 25
Back Stabilization		Back Stabilization	
Hip Routine		Hip Routine	

Strength Phase

Day 1		Day 3	
Rotator Cuff Warm-up	x 2	Rotator Cuff Warm-up	x 2
Push-ups	2 x 15	Decline Push-ups	1 x 20
Torso Twists	2 x 15	DB Side Bends	1 x 10
DB Bench Press	3 x 10	DB Incline Press	3 x 8
DB Lying Flys	3 x 10	DB Incline Flys	3 x 10
Upright Rows	3 x 10	DB Standing Military Press	3 x 8
DB Front Raises	3 x 12	DB Reverse Lateral Raises	3 x 10
Rear Deltoid Pull	3 x 10 SS	DB Shrugs	3 x 10 SS
DB Hammer Curls	2 x 10	Dips	3 x 10
DB Incline Curls	2 x 10	DB Curls	2 x 10
DB Tricep Extension	2 x 10 SS	Tricep Push-down	2 x 10 SS
Rice Routine		Rice Routine	
Abdominal #1		Abdominal #2	

Day 2		Day 4	
Rotator Cuff Warm-up	x 2	Rotator Cuff Warm-up	x 2
Pull-ups	1 x 8	Pull-ups	1 x 8
Twisting Back Extension	1 x 10	Good Mornings	1 x 15
Hang Cleans	3 x 8	Front Squat	3 x 10
Walking Lunges	2 x 8	Push Press	2 x 8
Leg Extensions, Single	2 x 10	Lateral Lunges	2 x 8
Leg Curls, Single	2 x 10	Leg Curls	2 x 10 SS
T-Bar Rows	3 x 8	DB One Arm Rows	3 x 8
Pull-overs	3 x 8	Lat Pull-downs	3 x 10
Seated Calves	2 x 25	Standing Calves, Single	2 x 25
Slide Board	2 x 30	Slide Board	2 x 30
Back Stabilization		Back Stabilization	
Hip Routine		Hip Routine	

Power Phase

Day 1		Day 3	
Rotator Cuff Warm-up	x 2	Rotator Cuff Warm-up	x 2
DB Lying Flys (Light)	2 x 15	DB Incline Flys (Light)	2 x 15

DB Bench Press	1 x 8, 2 x 6	Towel Pull-ups	2 x 5
UE Step-ups	3 x 10 SS	DB Incline Press	3 x 6
DB Standing Military	3 x 8	DB Upright Rows	3 x 8
DB Bent-over Front Raises	3 x 10	DB Reverse Lateral Raises	3 x 10
Bench Dips	2 x 15	Dips	2 x 12
DB Tricep Extension	3 x 8	Tricep Push-down	2 x 10
DB Hammer Curls	3 x 10 SS	DB Incline Curls	2 x 10 SS
Med Ball Abdominal		Abdominal #2	
Back Stabilization		Back Stabilization	
Plyometrics #'s	3, 32	Plyometrics #'s	11, 30

Day 2		Day 4	
Rotator Cuff Warm-up	x 2	Rotator Cuff Warm-up	x 2
Twisting Back Extension	2 x 15	DB Stiff Leg Dead Lift	2 x 15
Leg Extensions (Light)	2 x 15	Walking Lunges	2 x 10
Leg Curls (Light)	2 x 15 SS	Leg Curls	2 x 10 SS
Quarter Squat	3 x 8	Hang Cleans	3 x 5
Leg Sled	3 x 8	Push Press	3 x 5
DB Step-ups	2 x 8	Cross Over Lunges	3 x 8
Single Leg 6 Inch Box Jump	2 x 5 SS	Straight Bar Pull-downs	3 x 8
Seated Rows	3 x 10	Lat Pull-downs (ALT)	3 x 16
DB Pull-overs	4 x 8	Med Ball Routine #'s	9, 12
Med Ball Routine	5, 7	Slide Board	2 x 30

Peak/Transition Phase

Day 1		Day 3	
Rotator Cuff Warm-up	x 1	Rotator Cuff Warm-up	x 1
Med Ball Push-ups	1 x 10 (R/L)	Towel Pull-ups	1 x 10
DB Lying Flys (Light)	1 x 15	DB Incline Flys (Light)	1 x 15
DB Bench Press	1 x 8, 1 x 6, 1 x 4	DB Incline Press	3 x 8
Med Ball Over-head Pass	3 x 10 SS	UE Step-ups	3 x 10 SS
Upright Rows	3 x 8	DB Push Press	3 x 5
DB Front Raises	2 x 10	DB Bent-over Front Raises	2 x 10
DB Lateral Raises	2 x 10 SS	Rear Deltoid Pull	2 x 10 SS
Dips	2 x 10	Dips	1 x 10
Med Ball Abdominal		Abdominal #2	

Day 2		Day 4	
Rotator Cuff Warm-up	x 1	Rotator Cuff Warm-up	x 1
Twisting Back Extension	1 x 15	Good Mornings	1 x 20
Torso Twists	1 x 20	Torso Twists	1 x 20

Power Cleans	1 x 8, 1 x 6, 1 x 4	Leg Sled	1 x 8, 1 x 6, 1 x 4
Lateral Cone Hops	3 x 10 SS	Double Leg Bound	3 x 10 SS
Step-ups	2 x 8	Cross Over Lunges	2 x 8
Leg Curls	2 x 10 SS	Leg Curl	2 x 10 SS
DB One Arm Rows	3 x 8	Seated Row	3 x 8
Pull-overs	3 x 8	Straight Bar Pull-downs	3 x 8 SS
Back Stabilization		Back Stabilization	
Med Ball Routine #'s	5, 7	Slide Board	2 x 30

BASEBALL/SOFTBALL (IN-SEASON PHASE)

Day 1		Day 2	
Rotator Cuff Warm-up	x 2	Rotator Cuff Warm-up	x 2
Med Ball Push-ups	1 x 10	Towel Pull-ups	1 x 8
UE Step-ups	1 x 10	Good Mornings	1 x 15
DB Standing Military Press	3 x 8	Hang Cleans	2 x 8
Med Ball Over-head Pass	3 x 10 SS	Quarter Squat	2 x 8
DB Upright Rows	2 x 8	Pull-overs	3 x 8
Dips	2 x 10	Seated Calves	2 x 25
DB Hammer Curls	2 x 10	Abdominal #1	
Rice Routine		Back Stabilization	
Med Ball Abdominal		Hip Routine	

BASKETBALL

Introduction Phase

Day 1		Day 3	
Rotator Cuff Warm-up	x 2	Rotator Cuff Warm-up	x 2
Push-ups	1 x 10	Decline Push-ups	1 x 10
Bench Dips	1 x 10	Dips	1 x 8
Bench Press	3 x 12	DB Bench Press	3 x 12
Military Press	3 x 12	DB Incline Press	3 x 12
DB Lying Flys	3 x 15	DB Military Press	3 x 10
DB Upright Rows	3 x 15 SS	DB Front Raises	3 x 15
DB Reverse Lateral Raises	3 x 15	DB Lateral Raises	3 x 15 SS
Lying Tricep Extension	3 x 15	DB Tricep Extension	3 x 10

Straight Bar Curls	3 x 15 SS	DB Hammer Curls	3 x 10 SS
Rice Routine		Rice Routine	
Abdominals #1		Abdominals #2	

Day 2		Day 4	
Rotator Cuff Warm-up	x 1	Rotator Cuff Warm-up	x 1
Pull-ups	2 x 5	Pull-ups	2 x 5
Good Mornings	2 x 10 SS	DB Stiff Leg Dead Lift	2 x 10 SS
High Pulls	3 x 8	Power Squat	3 x 10
DB Hang Cleans	3 x 12	Hang Cleans	3 x 10
Leg Sled, Single	3 x 15	Leg Sled	3 x 12
Lat Pull-downs	3 x 15	Seated Rows	3 x 15
DB Pull-overs	3 x 15 SS	Lat Pull-downs	3 x 12
Leg Extensions	2 x 15	Walking Lunges	2 x 10
Leg Curl	2 x 15 SS	Leg Curls	2 x 15 SS
Back Stabilization		Back Stabilization	
Hip Routine		Hip Routine	

Strength Phase

Day 1		Day 3	
Rotator Cuff Warm-up	x 2	Rotator Cuff Warm-up	x 2
Incline Push-ups	2 x 15	Med Ball Push-ups	2 x 15
DB Incline Fly	2 x 15 SS	DB Lying Fly	2 x 10 SS
Bench Press	1 x 10, 2 x 8	DB Bench Press	3 x 8
Upright Rows	3 x 10	DB Incline Press	3 x 8
Rear Deltoid Pull	3 x 10	DB Push Press	2 x 8
DB Front Raises	3 x 10 SS	DB Front Raises	3 x 10
Dips	3 x 10	DB Lateral Raises	3 x 10 SS
Straight Bar Curls	3 x 10 SS	DB Tricep Extension	3 x 10
DB Incline Curls	3 x 10	DB Hammer Curls	3 x 10 SS
Rice Routine		Rice Routine	
Med Ball Abdominal		Abdominal #2	

Day 2		Day 4	
Rotator Cuff Warm-up	x 2	Rotator Cuff Warm-up	x 2
Pull-ups	2 x 8	Pull-ups	1 x 8
Good Mornings	2 x 10 SS	Twisting Back Extension	1 x 10
High Pulls	3 x 8	Front Squat	1 x 10, 2 x 8
DB Hang Cleans	3 x 8	Hang Cleans	2 x 8
Lat Pull-downs	3 x 10	Lat Pull-downs	3 x 16

T-Bar Rows	3 x 10		DB Pull-overs	3 x 10
Lateral Lunges	2 x 10		Leg Extensions, Single	2 x 12
Leg Curls	2 x 12 SS		Leg Curls, Single	2 x 12 SS
Standing Calves, Single	2 x 25		Seated Calves	2 x 25
Back Stabilization			Back Stabilization	
Hip Routine			Hip Routine	
Slide Board	2 x 30		Ladder	2 sets

Power Phase

Day 1

Rotator Cuff Warm-up	x 2
Push-ups	2 x 15
Bench Press	1 x 8, 2 x 6
DB Incline Press	1 x 8, 2 x 6
Med Ball Over-head Pass	3 x 10 SS
Military Press	3 x 8
Rear Deltoid Pulls	3 x 10
DB Upright Rows	3 x 10 SS
Dips	3 x 10
DB Seated Curls	3 x 10
Abdominal #1	
Plyometrics #'s	4, 6, 8, 9

Day 3

Rotator Cuff Warm-up	x 2
Decline Push-ups	2 x 10
DB Bench Press	3 x 6
Incline Press	3 x 8
Med Ball Chest Pass	3 x 10 SS
DB Push Press	3 x 8
DB Reverse Lateral Raises	3 x 10
DB Bent-over Front Raises	3 x 10 SS
DB Tricep Extension	3 x 8
DB Hammer Curls	3 x 10 SS
Abdominal #2	
Plyometrics #'s	7, 12, 14

Day 2

Rotator Cuff Warm-up	x 2
Torso Twists	2 x 10 SS
Good Mornings	2 x 10 SS
Pull-ups	2 x 8
Power Cleans	1 x 8, 2 x 6
Quarter Squat	3 x 8
Single Leg 6-Inch Box Jump	3 x 5 SS
Lateral Lunge	3 x 10
Lat Pull-down	3 x 10
DB Pull-over	3 x 10
Back Stabilization	
Med Ball Routine #'s	1, 4, 8
Slide Board	2 x 30

Day 4

Rotator Cuff Warm-up	x 2
Torso Twists	2 x 10 SS
DB Stiff Leg Dead Lift	2 x 10 SS
Pull-ups	2 x 8
Hang Cleans	3 x 6
Lateral Cone Hops	3 x 10 SS
Leg Extension	2 x 10
Leg Curls	2 x 10 SS
Seated Row	3 x 10
Lat Pull-down	3 x 10
Back Stabilization	
Hip Routine	
Ladder	2 sets

Peak/Transition Phase

Day 1	
Rotator Cuff Warm-up	x 2
DB Lying Flys	2 x 15
Bench Press	1 x 8, 1 x 6, 1 x 4
Med Ball Chest Pass	3 x 10 SS
Incline Press	3 x 6
DB Military Press	3 x 8
DB Upright Rows	3 x 10 SS
Dips	2 x 10
DB Seated Curls	2 x 10
Med Ball Abdominal	
Plyometrics #'s	17, 10, 12, 16

Day 3	
Rotator Cuff Warm-up	x 2
DB Incline Flys	2 x 15
DB Incline Press	1 x 8, 2 x 6
Med Ball Over-head Pass	3 x 10 SS
DB Push Press	2 x 6
Upright Rows	2 x 12
DB Bent-over Front Raises	2 x 10 SS
DB Tricep Extension	3 x 8
DB Hammer Curls	3 x 10 SS
Abdominal #2	
Plyometrics #'s	22, 23, 27, 29

Day 2	
Rotator Cuff Warm-up	x 2
Good Mornings	2 x 15
Power Cleans	1 x 8, 2 x 5
Lateral Cone Hops	3 x 10 SS
Leg Sled	1 x 10, 1 x 6, 1 x 4
Lat Pull-downs	2 x 10
Leg Extensions, Single	2 x 10
Leg Curls, Single	2 x 10
Standing Calves, Single	2 x 30
Back Stabilization	
Med Ball Routine #'s	7, 10, 15
Ladder	1 set

Day 4	
Rotator Cuff Warm-up	x 2
Good Mornings	2 x 15
Quarter Squat	1 x 8, 2 x 5
Squat Jumps	3 x 10 SS
Pull-overs	2 x 10
Seated Rows	2 x 10 SS
Lateral Lunges	2 x 8
Leg Curls	2 x 10 SS
Seated Calves	2 x 25
Back Stabilization	
Slide Board	2 x 20
Ladder	1 set

BASKETBALL (IN-SEASON PHASE)

Day 1	
Rotator Cuff Warm-up	
Push-ups	1 x 10
DB Tricep Extensions	1 x 15
DB Bench Press	3 x 8
Med Ball Chest Pass	3 x 10 SS
DB Upright Rows	2 x 10
Quarter Squat	3 x 8

Day 2	
Rotator Cuff Warm-up	
Towel Pull-ups	1 x 5
Decline Push-ups	1 x 10
Med Ball Over-head Pass	1 x 10
Hang Cleans	3 x 6
Ice Skaters	3 x 10 SS
DB Front Raises	2 x 15

Squat Jumps	3 x 10 SS		DB Bent-over Lateral Raises	2 x 15 SS
DB Pull-overs	2 x 10		Seated Rows	2 x 10
Med Ball Abdominal			DB Incline Hammer Curls	2 x 10
Hip Routine			Back Stabilization	
Ladder	1 Set		Slide Board	2 x 30

CREW

Introduction Phase

Day 1			Day 3	
Rotator Cuff Warm-up			Rotator Cuff Warm-up	
Push-ups	3 x 10		Incline Push-ups	3 x 15
DB Bench Press	3 x 15		DB Incline Press	3 x 15
DB Lying Flys	3 x 15		DB Incline Flys	3 x 15
DB Upright Rows	3 x 15		DB Front Raises	3 x 15
DB Bent-over Front Raises	3 x 15		DB Lateral Raises	3 x 15 SS
DB Bent-over Lateral Raises	3 x 15 SS		Rear Deltoid Pull	3 x 15
Dips	3 x 8		Bench Dips	3 x 10
Tricep Push-down	3 x 15		DB Tricep Kickback	3 x 10
DB Hammer Curls	3 x 10		DB Incline Curls	3 x 10
E-Z Bar Curls	3 x 15		Straight Bar Curls	3 x 12
Rice Routine			Rice Routine	
Abdominal #1			Abdominal #2	

Day 2			Day 4	
Rotator Cuff Warm-up	x 1		Rotator Cuff Warm-up	x 1
Towel Pull-ups	3 x 5		Pull-ups	3 x 5
Good Mornings	3 x 20		Back Extension	3 x 20
High Pulls	3 x 10		Hang Snatch	3 x 8
Hang Cleans	3 x 8		Power Shrug	3 x 8
Front Squat	2 x 10		Power Squat	3 x 12
Leg Curls	2 x 10 SS		Leg Curls	3 x 15 SS
Seated Calves	2 x 25		Standing Calves	2 x 30
T-Bar Rows	3 x 15		Seated Rows	3 x 15
DB One Arm Rows	3 x 10		Lat Pull-downs	3 x 15
Hip Routine			Hip Routine	
Back Stabilization			Back Stabilization	

Strength Phase

Day 1		Day 3	
Rotator Cuff Warm-up		Rotator Cuff Warm-up	
Incline Push-ups	3 x 15	Incline Push-ups	3 x 20
DB Bench Press	1 x 10, 3 x 8	DB Incline Press	1 x 10, 3 x 8
Cable Upright Rows	3 x 12	Cable Front Raises	3 x 12
DB Reverse Lateral Raises	3 x 12 SS	Cable Lateral Raises	3 x 12
DB Bent-over Lateral Raises	3 x 12	Rear Deltoid Pull	3 x 12
Dips	3 x 10	Bench Dips	3 x 15
Reverse Tricep Push-down	3 x 10	Tricep Push-down	3 x 10
DB Incline Hammer Curls	3 x 10 SS	DB Curls	3 x 10
Straight Bar Curls	3 x 10	E-Z Bar Curls	3 x 10
Rice Routine		Rice Routine	
Abdominal #1		Abdominal #2	

Day 2		Day 4	
Rotator Cuff Warm-up		Rotator Cuff Warm-up	
Towel Pull-ups	3 x 8	Pull-ups	3 x 8
Twisting Back Extension	3 x 10	Good Mornings	3 x 20
Torso Twists	3 x 20 SS	Torso Twists	3 x 20 SS
High Pulls	3 x 8	*Hang Clean Combo	2 x 6
Power Cleans	3 x 8	DB Squat	2 x 12
Walking Lunges	2 x 10	Leg Curls	2 x 12 SS
Leg Curls	2 x 10 SS	Standing Calves	3 x 35
Seated Calves	2 x 30	T-Bar Rows	3 x 10
Barbell Bent-over Rows	3 x 10	Lat Pull-downs	3 x 10
Straight Bar Lat Pull-downs	3 x 10	Hip Routine	
Hip Routine		Back Stabilization	
Back Stabilization			

*Hang Clean Combo: Perform hang clean, front squat, and push press for one repetition.

Power Phase

Day 1		Day 3	
Rotator Cuff Warm-up	x 1	Rotator Cuff Warm-up	x 1
Push-ups	3 x 15	Incline Push-ups	3 x 25
Back Extension	3 x 15 SS	Torso Twists	2 x 20
DB Bench Press	1 x 8, 3 x 6	DB Incline Press	1 x 8, 3 x 6
DB Lying Flys	2 x 10	DB Incline Flys	2 x 10
DB Upright Rows	3 x 10	DB Front Raises	3 x 10
DB Bent-over Front Raises	3 x 10 SS	DB Lateral Raises	3 x 10 TS

DB Bent-over Lateral Raises	3 x 10
E-Z Bar Curls	3 x 10
Dips	2 x 10
DB Hammer Curls	2 x 10
Abdominal #1	
Med Ball Routine #'s	2, 6, 12

Rear Deltoid Pull	3 x 10
Straight Bar Curls	3 x 10
Bench Dips	2 x 20
DB Curls	2 x 10 SS
Abdominal #2	
Med Ball Routine #'s	13, 14, 15

Day 2

Rotator Cuff Warm-up	x 1
Pull-ups	3 x 10
Twisting Back Extension	2 x 20
High Pulls	3 x 6
Power Cleans	1 x 8, 3 x 6
Double Leg Speed Hops	4 x 10 SS
DB Stiff Leg Dead Lift	2 x 10
Leg Curls	2 x 10 SS
DB One Arm Rows	3 x 10
Standing Lat Pull-downs	3 x 10
Hip Routine	
Back Stabilization	

Day 4

Rotator Cuff Warm-up	x 1
Pull-ups	3 x 10
Good Mornings	2 x 20
Hang Snatch	3 x 5
Power Squat	3 x 8
Box Jumps	3 x 30 SS
Leg Curls	2 x 10
Seated Rows	3 x 10
Lat Pull-downs	3 x 10
Standing Calves	2 x 40
Hip Routine	
Back Stabilization	

Peak/Transition Phase

Day 1

Rotator Cuff Warm-up	x 1
Push-ups	2 x 20
Torso Twists	2 x 20 SS
DB Bench Press	1 x 8, 1 x 6, 2 x 4
Med Ball Chest Pass	4 x 10 SS
Cable Front Raises	2 x 8
Cable Lateral Raises	2 x 8 SS
Rear Deltoid Pull	3 x 8
Dips	2 x 12
DB Incline Hammer Curls	2 x 10
Med Ball Abdominal	
Med Ball Routine #'s	2, 6, 12
Back Stabilization	

Day 3

Rotator Cuff Warm-up	x 1
Incline Push-ups	2 x 30
Torso Twists	2 x 20 SS
DB Incline Press	1 x 8, 1 x 6, 2 x 4
Med Ball Supine Drops	4 x 8 SS
Upright Rows	2 x 8
DB Bent-over Front Raises	3 x 8
DB Reverse Lateral Raises	3 x 8 SS
Bench Dips	2 x 20
Straight Bar Curls	2 x 10 SS
Abdominal #2	
Med Ball Routine #'s	1, 4
Back Stabilization	

Day 2

Rotator Cuff Warm-up	x 1
Towel Pull-ups	2 x 10
Twisting Back Extension	2 x 20 SS
Power Cleans	1 x 8, 1 x 6, 3 x 4

Day 4

Rotator Cuff Warm-up	x 1
Pull-ups	3 x 10
Good Mornings	3 x 20 SS
Squat	1 x 8, 1 x 6, 2 x 4

Leg Sled	1 x 8, 1 x 6, 2 x 4	Squat Jumps	4 x 10 SS
Ankle Hops	4 x 8 SS	Hang Cleans	3 x 5
Step-ups	2 x 8	Leg Extensions	2 x 10
Leg Curls	2 x 10 SS	Leg Curls	2 x 10 SS
Barbell Bent-over Rows	3 x 8	T-Bar Rows	3 x 8
Lat Pull-downs	3 x 10	Straight Bar Lat Pull-downs	3 x 10
Box Jumps	3 x 30	Box Jumps	2 x 45

CREW (IN SEASON PHASE)

Day 1		Day 2	
Rotator Cuff Warm-up		Rotator Cuff Warm-up	
Towel Pull-ups	2 x 5	Incline Push-ups	2 x 15
Back Extension	2 x 10 SS	Med Ball Chest Pass	2 x 10 SS
DB Bench Press	3 x 8	High Pulls	2 x 8
DB Lying Flys	3 x 12	Double Leg Speed Hops	2 x 10 SS
Cable Upright Row	2 x 10	Barbell Bent-over Row	3 x 10
Rear Deltoid Pull	2 x 12 SS	DB Bent-over Front Raise	3 x 12 SS
Hang Cleans	3 x 8	DB Squat	2 x 12
Squat Jumps	3 x 10 SS	BOX x Jumps	2 x 10 SS
Dips	2 x 10	Bench Dips	2 x 20
DB Incline Hammer Curl	3 x 12	Straight Bar Curl	3 x 12
Abdominal #1		Med Ball Abdominal	
Back Stabilization		Back Stabilization	

CROSS COUNTRY/TRACK (DISTANCE)

Introduction Phase

Day 1		Day 3	
Rotator Cuff Warm-up	x 1	Rotator Cuff Warm-up	x 1
Push-ups	3 x 10	Incline Push-ups	3 x 15
DB Lying Flys	3 x 15	Dips	3 x 10
Leg Extensions	3 x 15	Tricep Push-down	3 x 15
Leg Curls	3 x 15 SS	Step-ups	3 x 10
DB Upright Rows	3 x 15	Leg Curls	3 x 15 SS
DB Lateral Raises	3 x 12 SS	DB Hammer Curls	3 x 10

DB Tricep Kickback	3 x 12	DB Front Raises	3 x 12
DB Incline Hammer Curls	3 x 10	Rear Deltoid Pull	3 x 10 SS
Abdominal #1		Med Ball Abdominal	
Back Stabilization		Back Stabilization	
Hip Routine		Hip Routine	

Day 2

Pull-ups	3 x 8
Rotator Cuff Warm-up	x 1
DB Squat	3 x 15
Lunges	3 x 15
Seated Rows	3 x 12
DB Curls	3 x 12
Bench Dips	3 x 20
DB Reverse Lateral Raises	3 x 12
DB Bent-over Lateral Raises	3 x 12 SS
Abdominal #2	
Back Stabilization	
Hip Routine	

Strength Phase

Day 1		Day 3	
Rotator Cuff Warm-up	x 1	Rotator Cuff Warm-up	x 1
Push-ups	3 x 15	Incline Push-ups	2 x 20
DB Incline Press	3 x 10	Dips	2 x 12
DB Incline Flys	3 x 10	Power Squat	3 x 10
DB Squat	2 x 10	Lunge Squat	3 x 10
Leg Curls	2 x 10 SS	Leg Curls, Single	3 x 15
DB Reverse Lateral Raises	3 x 10	Straight Bar Curls	2 x 12
DB Bent-over Lateral Raises	3 x 10 SS	Abdominal #2	
Abdominal #1		Back Stabilization	
Back Stabilization		Hip Routine	
Hip Routine			

Day 2

Rotator Cuff Warm-up	x 1
Pull-ups	3 x 10
Walking Lunges	3 x 10
DB Stiff Leg Dead Lift	3 x 10 TS
Leg Curls	3 x 10

Seated Rows	3 x 10
Lat Pull-downs	3 x 10
Seated Calves	2 x 25
Med Ball Abdominal	
Back Stabilization	
Hip Routine	

Power Phase

Day 1

Rotator Cuff Warm-up	x 1
Push-ups	3 x 15
Back Extension	3 x 15 SS
DB Incline Flys	3 x 15
DB Bench Press	3 x 8
DB Squat	3 x 8
Squat Jumps	3 x 10 SS
Cable Front Raises	3 x 10
Cable Lateral Raises	3 x 10 TS
DB Bent-over Lateral Raises	3 x 10
Abdominal #1	
Hip Routine	
Back Stabilization	

Day 2

Rotator Cuff Warm-ups	x 1
Pull-ups	3 x 10
Good Mornings	3 x 10 TS
Torso Twists	3 x 20
Lunges	2 x 10
Single Lateral Cone Hops	2 x 10 SS
Leg Extensions, Single	2 x 10
Leg Curls, Single	2 x 10
Seated Rows	3 x 10
Abdominal #2	
Back Stabilization	

Day 3

Rotator Cuff Warm-up	x 1
Push-ups	3 x 15
Twisting Back Extension	3 x 15 SS
Dips	2 x 12
DB Step-ups	2 x 10
Single Leg Speed Hops	2 x 10 SS
DB Incline Hammer Curls	3 x 10
E-Z Bar Curls	3 x 10
DB Tricep Kickback	3 x 10
Med Ball Abdominal	
Hip Routine	
Back Stabilization	
Plyometrics #'s	2, 3, 26

Peak/Transition Phase

Day 1

Decline Push-ups	3 x 10
DB Lying Flys	3 x 10 SS

Day 3

Incline Push-ups	3 x 20
Bench Dips	3 x 20

DB Upright Rows	2 x 10	DB Hammer Curls	3 x 10
DB Lateral Raises	2 x 10	Tricep Push-down	3 x 10
Rear Deltoid Pull	2 x 10 SS	E-Z Bar Curls	3 x 10
Walking Lunges	2 x 10	Seated Rows	3 x 10
Alt Scissor Jumps	2 x 10 SS	Lat Pull-downs	3 x 12
Abdominal #1		Med Ball Abdominal	
Plyometrics #'s	1, 9, 10	Plyometrics #'s	18, 20, 26

Day 2

Rotator Cuff Warm-up	x 1
Pull-ups	3 x 10
Torso Twists	3 x 20 SS
Quarter Squat	3 x 8
Single Leg 6-Inch Box Jumps	3 x 10 SS
Leg Extensions	2 x 10
Leg Curls	2 x 10 SS
Back Stabilization	
Hip Routine	

CROSS COUNTRY/TRACK (DISTANCE) (IN SEASON PHASE)

Day 1

Rotator Cuff Warm-up	x 1
Pull-ups	2 x 8
Good Mornings	2 x 15 SS
Quarter Squat	2 x 12
Squat Jumps	2 x 10 SS
Cable Upright Rows	3 x 15
DB Lateral Raises	3 x 15 SS
DB Incline Hammer Curls	3 x 12
Dips	3 x 10
Abdominal #1	
Back Stabilization	

Day 2

Rotator Cuff Warm-up	x 1
Push-ups	2 x 15
Twisting Back Extension	2 x 10 SS
Walking Lunges	3 x 10
Alt Scissor Jumps	3 x 10 SS
DB Front Raises	2 x 15
DB Bent-over Lateral Raises	2 x 15 SS
Cable Curls	2 x 10
Bench Dips	2 x 20
Med Ball Abdominal	
Hip Routine	

DIVING/GYMNASTICS

Introduction Phase

Day 1

| Rotator Cuff Warm-up | x 2 |

Day 3

| Rotator Cuff Warm-up | x 2 |

Push-ups	3 x 10	Decline Push-ups	3 x 10
Dips	3 x 10	Dips	3 x 10
DB Standing Military Press	3 x 15	Upright Rows	3 x 15
DB Bent-over Front Raises	3 x 15	Cable Front Raises	3 x 15
Rear Deltoid Pull	3 x 15	Cable Lateral Raises	3 x 15
Straight Bar Curls	3 x 10	DB Incline Curls	3 x 10
DB Hammer Curls	3 x 10	Cable Curls	3 x 10
DB Lying Tricep Extension	3 x 15	DB Tricep Extension	3 x 15
Abdominal #1		Med Ball Abdominal	

Day 2		**Day 4**	
Rotator Cuff Warm-up	x 1	Rotator Cuff Warm-up	x 1
Pull-ups	3 x 5	Incline Pull-ups	3 x 10
Twisting Back Extension	3 x 10 SS	Back Extension	3 x 10
High Pulls	3 x 12	Push Press	3 x 10
Hang Cleans	2 x 10	Power Squat	3 x 10
Walking Lunges	3 x 20	Reverse Lunges	3 x 10
Stiff Leg Dead Lift	3 x 10 SS	Leg Curls	3 x 10 SS
Barbell Bent-over Rows	2 x 15	Straight Lat Pull-downs	2 x 15
Standing Calves	2 x 30	Seated Calves	2 x 25
Hip Routine		Hip Routine	
Back Stabilization		Back Stabilization	

Strength Phase

Day 1		**Day 3**	
Rotator Cuff Warm-up	x 2	Rotator Cuff Warm-up	x 2
Push-ups	3 x 12	Decline Push-ups	3 x 12
Dips	3 x 12	Dips	3 x 12
DB Incline Flys	3 x 10	DB Lying Flys	3 x 10
DB Bent-over Front Raises	3 x 12	Cable Front Raises	3 x 12
Rear Deltoid Pull	3 x 12	Cable Lateral Raises	3 x 12 SS
Straight Bar Curls	3 x 10	DB Incline Curls	3 x 10
DB Hammer Curls	3 x 10	Cable Curls	3 x 10
Abdominal #1		Med Ball Abdominal	

Day 2		**Day 4**	
Rotator Cuff Warm-up	x 1	Rotator Cuff Warm-up	x 1
Pull-ups	3 x 8	Towel Pull-ups	3 x 8
Twisting Back Extension	3 x 12 SS	Back Extension	3 x 15
High Pulls	3 x 10	Push Press	3 x 8
Hang Cleans	2 x 8	Lateral Lunges	3 x 10
Quarter Squat	3 x 10	Double Leg Speed Hops	3 x 10 SS
Squat Jumps	3 x 10 SS	Leg Curls, Single	3 x 10

Standing Calves, Single	2 x 40		Seated Calves	3 x 30
Hip Routine			Hip Routine	
Back Stabilization				

Power Phase

Day 1			Day 3	
Rotator Cuff Warm-up	x 2		Rotator Cuff Warm-up	x 2
Push-ups	3 x 15		Decline Push-ups	3 x 15
Dips	3 x 15		Dips	3 x 15
Med Ball Chest Pass	3 x 10 SS		Med Ball Over-head Pass	3 x 10 SS
DB Lying Flys	3 x 10		DB Bent-over Front Raise	3 x 10
Upright Rows	3 x 10		Cable Front Raise	3 x 10
DB Bent-over Lateral Raises	3 x 10		Cable Lateral Raise	3 x 10 SS
Straight Bar Curls	3 x 8		DB Incline Curls	3 x 8
Abdominal #1			Med Ball Abdominal	
Plyometrics #'s	2, 4, 7, 8		Plyometrics #'s	11, 12, 27

Day 2			Day 4	
Rotator Cuff Warm-up	x 1		Rotator Cuff Warm-up	x 1
Pull-ups	3 x 10		Incline Pull-ups	3 x 10
Twisting Back Extension	3 x 20 SS		Back Extension	3 x 20
Power Cleans	3 x 8		Push Press	1 x 8, 1 x 6, 1 x 4
Alt Scissor Jumps	3 x 10 SS		DB Squat	3 x 10
Quarter Squat	3 x 10		Walking Lunges	3 x 10
Leg Curls	3 x 10 SS		Leg Curls	3 x 10 SS
Standing Calves, Single	2 x 30		Seated Calves	3 x 30
Hip Routine			Hip Routine	
Back Stabilization			Back Stabilization	
Med Ball Routine #'s	2, 12, 14		Med Ball Routine #'s 11, 13, 16	

Peak/Transition Phase

Day 1			Day 3	
Rotator Cuff Warm-up	x 2		Rotator Cuff Warm-up	x 2
Med Ball Push-ups	2 x 15		Decline Push-ups	2 x 15
Dips	2 x 15		Dips	3 x 15
UE Step-ups	3 x 10		Med Ball Chest Pass	3 x 10 SS
Med Ball Prone Push	3 x 10 SS		DB Bent-over Front Raises	2 x 10
Upright Rows	3 x 8		Cable Front Raises	2 x 10 TS
Rear Deltoid Pull	3 x 10		Cable Lateral Raises	2 x 10
DB Hammer Curls	3 x 8		Cable Curls	3 x 8

Abdominal #1		Abdominal #2	
Plyometrics #'s	1, 3, 5, 10	Plyometrics#'S	11, 19, 22, 23

Day 2		Day 4	
Rotator Cuff Warm-up	x 1	Rotator Cuff Warm-up	x 1
Pull-ups	2 x 10	Incline Pull-ups	3 x 10
Twisting Back Extension	2 x 20 SS	Back Extension	3 x 20
Power Cleans	3 x 8	Push Press	1 x 8, 1 x 5, 1 x 3
Single Leg 6-Inch Box Jumps	3 x 10 SS	Quarter Squat	1 x 8,1 x 6, 1 x 4
Leg Extension	2 x 10	Lateral Cone Hops	3 x 10 SS
Leg Curls	2 x 10 SS	Leg Curls	2 x 10
Standing Calves	2 x 30	Seated Calves	2 x 30 SS
Hip Routine		Hip Routine	
Back Stabilization		Back Stabilization	
Med Ball Routine #'s	5, 11, 12	Med Ball Routine #'s	15, 16

DIVING/GYMNASTICS (IN-SEASON PHASE)

Day 1		Day 2	
Rotator Cuff Warm-up	x 2	Rotator Cuff Warm-up	
Decline Push-ups	2 x 10	Pull-ups	2 x 10
Med Ball Supine Drops	2 x 10 SS	Incline Pull-ups	2 x 10
DB Incline Fly	3 x 12	Hang Cleans	3 x 8
DB Standing Military Press	3 x 8	Box Jumps	3 x 10 SS
Rear Deltoid Pull	3 x 10 SS	DB Squat	2 x 10
DB Hammer Curls	2 x 10	Double Leg Speed Hops	2 x 10 SS
Dips	2 x 10	Seated Calves	2 x 25
Abdominal #1		Med Ball Abdominal	
Back Stabilization		Hip Routine	

FOOTBALL/RUGBY (KICKERS)

Introduction Phase

Day 1		Day 3	
Rotator Cuff Warm-up	x 1	Rotator Cuff Warm-up	x 1
Good Mornings	2 x 15	Good Mornings	2 x 15

Torso Twists	2 x 20 TS	Torso Twists	2 x 20 TS
Pull-ups	2 x 8	Incline Pull-ups	2 x 10
DB Squat	3 x 15	Leg Sled, Single	3 x 15
DB Hang Cleans	3 x 10	Leg Curls	3 x 15 SS
Step-ups	3 x 10	Lunges (4-Way)	3 x 5
Straight Lat Pull-downs	3 x 15	DB One Arm Rows	3 x 10
Seated Rows	3 x 15	Lat Pull-downs	3 x 15
Abdominal #1		Abdominal #2	

Day 2		**Day 4**	
Rotator Cuff Warm-up	x 1	Rotator Cuff Warm-up	x 1
Incline Push-ups	3 x 20	Decline Push-ups	3 x 15
Twisting Back Extension	3 x 20 SS	Back Extension	3 x 10 SS
DB Lying Flys	3 x 15	Military Press	3 x 10
DB Bench Press	3 x 12	DB Front Raises	3 x 15
DB Incline Press	3 x 15	DB Lateral Raises	3 x 15 SS
Dips	3 x 10	DB Hammer Curls	3 x 10
DB Tricep Extension	3 x 15	DB Seated Curls	3 x 10
Hip Routine		Hip Routine	
Back Stabilization		Back Stabilization	

Strength Phase

Day 1		**Day 3**	
Rotator Cuff Warm-up	x 1	Rotator Cuff Warm-up	x 1
Good Mornings	2 x 15	Good Mornings	2 x 15
Torso Twists	2 x 20 TS	Torso Twists	2 x 20 TS
Pull-ups	2 x 10	Incline Pull-ups	2 x 10
DB Squat	3 x 10	Hang Snatch	3 x 8
DB Hang Cleans	3 x 10	Leg Extensions	3 x 10
Lunges (4-Way)	3 x 5	Leg Curls	3 x 10 SS
Straight Lat Pull-downs	3 x 12	DB One Arm Rows	3 x 10
Seated Rows	3 x 12	Lat Pull-downs	3 x 12
Abdominal #1		Med Ball Abdominal	

Day 2		**Day 4**	
Rotator Cuff Warm-up	x 1	Rotator Cuff Warm-up	x 1
Incline Push-ups	3 x 20	Decline Push-ups	3 x 15
Twisting Back Extension	3 x 20 SS	Back Extension	3 x 15 SS
DB Lying Flys	3 x 12	Military Press	3 x 8
Bench Press	3 x 10	Upright Rows	3 x 10
Incline Press	3 x 10	DB Bent-over Lateral Raises	3 x 10 SS
Bench Dips	3 x 15	DB Hammer Curls	3 x 10
DB Lying Tricep Extension	3 x 15	Straight Bar Curls	3 x 10

Hip Routine
Back Stabilization

Hip Routine
Back Stabilization

Power Phase

Day 1		Day 3	
Rotator Cuff Warm-up		Rotator Cuff Warm-up	
Pull-ups	2 x 10	Incline Pull-ups	2 x 10
Back Extensions	2 x 15 TS	Twisting Back Extension	2 x 20 TS
Torso Twists	2 x 20	DB Side Bends	2 x 10
Hang Cleans	4 x 6	Power Cleans	1 x 6, 3 x 4
Box Jumps	4 x 20 SS	Single Leg Speed Hop	4 x 10 SS
Quarter Squats	3 x 8	Walking Lunges	3 x 8
Step-ups	3 x 8	Lateral Lunges	3 x 8
Seated Row	3 x 10	Lat Pull-down	3 x 10
Straight Lat Pull-down	3 x 10	Pull-over	3 x 10
Med Ball Abdominal		Abdominal #2	
Plyometrics #'s	1, 3, 9	Plyometrics #'s	10, 18, 20

Day 2		Day 4	
Rotator Cuff Warm-up	x 1	Rotator Cuff Warm-up	x 1
Push-ups	2 x 15	Decline Push-ups	2 x 15
Torso Twists	2 x 20 SS	Torso Twists	2 x 20 SS
DB Bench Press	1 x 8, 1 x 6, 1 x 4	DB Military Press	1 x 8, 1 x 6, 1 x 4
DB Lying Flys	3 x 8	DB Upright Rows	3 x 8
DB Tricep Extension	3 x 8	Straight Bar Curls	3 x 10
DB Lying Tricep Extension	3 x 10	DB Incline Curls	3 x 10
Hip Routine		Back Stabilization	

Peak/Transition Phase

Day 1		Day 3	
Rotator Cuff Warm-up	x 1	Rotator Cuff Warm-up	
Pull-ups	1 x 10	Incline Pull-ups	1 x 10
Back ExtensionS	1 x 15	Twisting Back Extension	1 x 20
Torso Twists	1 x 20	DB Side Bends	1 x 10
Hang Cleans	3 x 5	Power Cleans	3 x 5
Box Jumps	3 x 10 SS	Single Leg Speed Hops	3 x 10 SS
Quarter Squats	3 x 8	Walking Lunges	2 x 8
Seated Rows	2 x 10	Lat Pull-downs	2 x 10
Straight Lat Pull-downs	2 x 10	Pull-overs	2 x 10
Med Ball Abdominal		Abdominal #2	
Plyometrics #'s	1, 3, 9	Plyometrics #'s	10, 18, 26

Day 2			Day 4		
Rotator Cuff Warm-up	x 1		Rotator Cuff Warm-up	x 1	
Push-ups	2 x 15		Decline Push-ups	2 x 15	
Torso Twists	2 x 20 SS		Torso Twists	2 x 20 SS	
Bench Press	1 x 8, 1 x 6, 1 x 4		Military Press	1 x 8, 1 x 6, 1 x 4	
Incline Press	3 x 5		DB Bent-over Lateral Raises	3 x 8	
Tricep Push-down	3 x 8		E-Z Bar Curls	3 x 10	
DB Lying Tricep Extension	3 x 10		DB Incline Hammer Curls	3 x 10	
Hip Routine					

FOOTBALL/RUGBY
(LINEBACKERS, TIGHT ENDS, AND FORWARDS)

Introduction Phase

Day 1		Day 3	
Rotator Cuff Warm-up	x 1	Rotator Cuff Warm-up	x 1
Push-ups	2 x 10	Decline Push-UPS	2 x 10
Neck (4-Way)	2 x 10 SS	Neck (4-Way)	2 x 10 SS
Bench Press (50%, 60%, 72.5%)	3 x 10	DB Bench Press	3 x 12
Incline Press	4 x 12	DB Incline Press	3 x 12
Rear Military	3 x 10	Military Press	4 x 10
Upright Rows	3 x 10 SS	DB Upright Rows	4 x 12
DB Lying Tricep Extension	3 x 10	DB Bent-over Lateral Raise	3 x 15
Dips	2 x 10	Bench Dips	3 x 20
DB Tricep Extension	3 x 10	Tricep Push-down	3 x 15
Wrist Flexion	2 x 20	Wrist Extension	2 x 20
Abdominal #1		Abdominal #2	

Day 2		Day 4	
Rotator Cuff Warm-up	x 1	Rotator Cuff Warm-up	x 1
Pull-ups	2 x 5	Pull-ups	2 x 5
Good Mornings	2 x 15 TS	Good Mornings	2 x 15 TS
DB Stiff Leg Dead Lift	2 x 12	Torso Twists	2 x 20
Hang Cleans	3 x 8	Hang Snatch	3 x 10
Dead Lift	4 x 10	Front Squat	3 x 10
Power Squat	3 x 10	Barbell Bent-over Rows	4 x 15
Lat Pull-downs	3 x 15	T-Bar Rows	3 x 10
Seated Rows	3 x 15	DB Pull-overs	3 x 12

Straight Bar Curls	3 x 15	Leg Extensions, Single	3 x 15
DB Hammer Curls	3 x 12	Leg Curls, Single	3 x 15
Hip Routine		Hip Routine	
Back Stabilization		Back Stabilization	

Strength Phase

Day 1		Day 3	
Rotator Cuff Warm-up	x 1	Rotator Cuff Warm-up	x 1
Neck (4-Way)	2 x 10	Neck (4-Way)	2 x 10
DB Lying Flys (Light)	2 x 15	Decline Push-ups	2 x 20
Bench Press	3 x 8	DB Bench Press	3 x 8
Incline Press	1 x 8, 3 x 6	DB Incline Press	1 x 8, 2 x 6
DB Military	4 x 8	Rear Military	1 x 8, 3 x 6
DB Front Raises	3 x 10	DB Upright Rows	3 x 10
DB Lateral Raises	3 x 10 SS	DB Reverse Lateral Raises	3 x 10 TS
Tricep Push-down	3 x 10	DB Bent-over Front Raises	3 x 10
Dips	3 x 10	DB Tricep Extension	3 x 8
DB Lying Tricep Extension	2 x 10	Bench Dips	3 x 10
Wrist Flexion	2 x 20	Wrist Extension	2 x 20
Abdominal #1		Abdominal #2	
Ladder	1 Set	Ladder	1 Set

Day 2		Day 4	
Rotator Cuff Warm-up	x 1	Rotator Cuff Warm-up	x 1
Back Extensions	2 x 15	Back Extensions	2 x 15
Torso Twists	2 x 20 TS	Torso Twists	2 x 20 TS
Prone Neck Extensions	2 x 30	Supine Neck Flexion	2 x 30
Power Cleans	3 x 6	Hang Snatch	3 x 8
Dead Lift	1 x 8, 2 x 6	Front Squat	3 x 8
Leg Sled	4 x 8	Power Shrugs	4 x 8
Seated Rows	3 x 10	Lat Pull-downs	3 x 16
T-Bar RowS	3 x 8	DB One Arm Rows	3 x 10
DB Incline Curls	3 x 10	Leg Extensions	2 x 15
Cable Curls	3 x 10	Leg Curls	2 x 15 SS
Seated Calves	2 x 25	Seated Calves	2 x 25
Hip Routine		Hip Routine	
Back Stabilization		Back Stabilization	
Slide Board	2 x 30	Slide Board	2 x 45

Power Phase

Day 1

Rotator Cuff Warm-up	x 1
Neck (4-Way)	2 x 10
UE Step-ups	2 x 10
Bench Press	1 x 8, 3 x 6
Incline Press	4 x 6
Med Ball Chest Pass	4 x 10 SS
Rear Military Press	3 x 6
Upright Rows	3 x 8
Dips	3 x 12
DB Lying Tricep Extension	3 x 10
Med Ball Abdominal	
Ladder	2 sets
Plyometrics #'s	1, 8, 11, 12

Day 3

Rotator Cuff Warm-up	x 1
Prone Neck Extensions	2 x 40
Decline Push-ups	2 x 10
DB Bench Press	3 x 6
DB Incline Press	3 x 6
DB Military Press	4 x 8
DB Front Raises	3 x 10
DB Lateral Raises	3 x 10 SS
Tricep Push-downs	3 x 10
DB Tricep Extension	3 x 10
Abdominal #2	
Ladder	2 sets
Plyometrics #'s	14, 16, 22, 23, 27

Day 2

Rotator Cuff Warm-up	x 1
Good Mornings	2 x 15
Pull-ups	2 x 8
*Power Clean Combo	3 x 5
Power Squat	1 x 8, 3 x 6
Lunges	3 x 8
Leg Curls	3 x 10 SS
Lat Pull-downs	3 x 12
T-Bar Rows	3 x 8
Seated Calves	2 x 30
Back Stabilization	
Med Ball Routine #'s	2, 6, 12, 13

Day 4

Rotator Cuff Warm-up	x 1
Twisting Back Extensions	2 x 20
Incline Pull-ups	2 x 10
Hang Snatch	2 x 8
Leg Sled	1 x 8, 3 x 5
Lateral Box Jumps	4 x 10 SS
Straight Lat Pull-downs	3 x 12
Seated Rows	3 x 8 SS
Barbell Bent-over Rows	3 x 10
Standing Calves, Single	2 x 30
Hip Routine	
Med Ball Routine #'s	11, 14, 15, 16

*Power Clean Combo: Perform power clean, front squat

Peak/Transition Phase

Day 1

Rotator Cuff Warm-up	x 1
Neck (4-Way)	2 x 10
DB Lying Fly (Light)	2 x 15
Bench Press	1 x 8, 1 x 6, 2 x 4
Incline Press	1 x 8, 1 x 6, 2 x 4
Med Ball Chest Pass	4 x 10
DB Incline Flys	3 x 8

Day 3

Rotator Cuff Warm-up	x 1
Neck (4-Way)	2 x 10
DB Incline Flys (Light)	2 x 15
DB Bench Press	3 x 6
Med Ball Over-head Pass	3 x 10 SS
DB Incline Press	3 x 6
Rear Military	3 x 5

DB Military Press	3 x 6	DB Upright Row	3 x 8
Upright Rows	3 x 8	DB Bent-over Front Raise	3 x 10
DB Tricep Extension	3 x 8	DB Bent-over Lateral Raise	3 x 10 SS
Dips	2 x 15	Dips	2 x 10
Rice Routine		Rice Routine	
Abdominal #1		Abdominal #2	
Ladder	1 set	Ladder	1 set
Plyometrics #'S	20, 21 (add sprint), 26	Plyometrics #'S	1, 7, 15, 21

Day 2		**Day 4**	
Rotator Cuff Warm-up	x 1	Rotator Cuff Warm-up	x 1
Good Mornings	2 x 15	Good Mornings	2 x 15
Supine Neck Flexion	2 x 30 SS	Prone Neck Extension	2 x 30 SS
Pull-ups	1 x 10	Incline Pull-ups	1 x 15
Power Cleans	1 x 8, 1 x 6, 1 x 4	Hang Snatch	2 x 8
Leg Sled	1 x 10, 1 x 5, 2 x 3	Power Squat	1 x 8, 3 x 5
Double Leg Speed Hops	4 x 10 SS	Lateral Cone Hops	4 x 10 SS
T-Bar Rows	3 x 8	Lat Pull-downs	3 x 10
DB Pull-over	3 x 8 SS	Seated Rows	3 x 8 SS
DB Incline Hammer Curls	3 x 10	Straight Bar Curls	3 x 10
E-Z Bar Curls	2 x 12	DB Hammer Curls	2 x 12
Back Stabilization		Hip Routine	
Med Ball Routine #'s	4, 6, 14, 15	Med Ball Routine #'s	5, 10, 12, 16

FOOTBALL/RUGBY (LINEMEN)

Introduction Phase

Day 1		**Day 3**	
Rotator Cuff Warm-up		Rotator Cuff Warm-up	x 1
Push-ups	2 x 10	Incline Push-up	2 x 20
Torso Twists	2 x 20 SS	Torso Twists	2 x 20 SS
Bench Press	1 x 10, 3 x 10	DB Bench Press	3 x 12
Incline Press	4 x 10	Close Grip Bench Press	3 x 10
DB Incline Flys	3 x 15	Military Press	3 x 10
DB Front Raises	3 x 15	Upright Rows	3 x 15
DB Lateral Raises	3 x 15 SS	DB Bent-over Lateral Raises	3 x 15
DB Lying Tricep Extension	3 x 15	DB Tricep Extension	3 x 12
Tricep Push-down	3 x 15	Reverse Tricep Push-down	3 x 15
Wrist Flexion	2 x 20	Wrist Extension	2 x 20
Abdominal #1		Abdominal #2	

Day 2	
Rotator Cuff Warm-up	x 1
Neck (4-Way)	1 x 10
Pull-ups	2 x 5
Good Mornings	2 x 15 SS
High Pulls	3 x 10
Hang Cleans	3 x 8
Power Shrugs	3 x 15
T-Bar Rows	3 x 15
Pull-overs	3 x 15
Lunges	3 x 10
Leg Curls	3 x 15 SS
Seated Calves	2 x 25
DB Incline Curls	3 x 10
Straight Bar Curls	3 x 12
Hip Routine	
Back Stabilization	

Day 4	
Rotator Cuff Warm-up	x 1
Neck (4-Way)	1 x 10
Incline Pull-ups	2 x 10
Stiff Leg Dead Lift	2 x 15 SS
Hang Snatch	2 x 8
Power Squat	3 x 10
Leg Sled	3 x 10
Leg Curls	3 x 15 SS
DB One Arm Rows	3 x 15
Straight Pulldowns	3 x 15
Lat Pull-downs	3 x 15
Standing Calves, Single	3 x 25
DB Incline Hammer Curls	3 x 10
Cable Curls	3 x 12
Hip Routine	
Back Stabilization	

Strength Phase

Day 1	
Rotator Cuff Warm-up	x 1
Prone Neck Extension	1 x 30
Push-ups	2 x 15
Torso Twists	2 x 20 SS
Bench Press	1 x 8, 3 x 8
Incline Press	3 x 10
Close Grip Incline Press	3 x 10
DB Standing Military Press	3 x 10
DB Bent-over Front Raises	3 x 10
DB Reverse Lateral Raises	3 x 10 SS
Dips	3 x 10
DB Tricep Extension	3 x 8
Rice Routine	
Abdominal #1	

Day 3	
Rotator Cuff Warm-up	x 1
Supine Neck Flexion	1 x 30
Close Grip Push-ups	2 x 15
Torso Twists	2 x 20 SS
Close Grip Bench Press	3 x 8
DB Incline Press	3 x 8
DB Incline Flys	3 x 10
Rear Military Press	3 x 8
DB Upright Rows	3 x 10
DB Front Raises	3 x 10 SS
Tricep Push-down	3 x 10
DB Lying Tricep Extension	3 x 10
Rice Routine	
Abdominal #2	

Day 2	
Rotator Cuff Warm-up	x 1
Neck (4-Way)	1 x 10
Pull-ups	2 x 8
Good Mornings	2 x 20 SS
High Pulls	2 x 8
Power Cleans	3 x 8

Day 4	
Rotator Cuff Warm-up	x 1
Neck (4-Way)	1 x 10
Incline Pull-ups	2 x 12
Good Mornings	2 x 20 SS
Dead Lift	3 x 8
Power Squat	1 x 10, 3 x 8

Power Shrugs	3 x 8	Leg Extensions	3 x 10
Leg Sled	4 x 8	Leg Curls	3 x 10 SS
Stiff Leg Dead Lift	4 x 10 SS	Seated Rows	3 x 10
T-Bar Rows	3 x 8	Lat Pull-downs	3 x 12
Close Grip Pull-downs	3 x 10	DB One Arm Rows	3 x 10
DB Curls	3 x 10	Straight Bar Curls	3 x 10
DB Hammer Curls	3 x 8	E-Z Bar Curls	3 x 8
Seated Calves	2 x 20	Seated Calves	2 x 20
Hip Routine		Hip Routine	
Back Stabilization		Back Stabilization	

Power Phase

Day 1		Day 3	
Rotator Cuff Warm-up	x 1	Rotator Cuff Warm-up	
Prone Neck Extension	1 x 30	Supine Neck Flexion	1 x 30
Push-ups	2 x 30	Close Grip Push-ups	2 x 15
DB Lying Flys (Light)	2 x 15 SS	DB Incline Flys (Light)	2 x 15 SS
Bench Press	1 x 8, 3 x 5	Close Grip Bench Press	4 x 6
Incline Press	1 x 8, 1 x 6, 2 x 4	DB Incline Press	3 x 6
Military Press	1 x 8, 2 x 6	DB Standing Military	3 x 10
Cable Front Raise	3 x 10	DB Reverse Lateral Raises	3 x 10
Cable Lateral Raise	3 x 10 SS	DB Bent-over Lateral Raises	3 x 10 SS
Dips	3 x 10	DB Tricep Extension	3 x 8
Tricep Push-down	3 x 10	DB Lying Tricep Extension	3 x 8
Abdominal #1		Med Ball Abdominal	
Ladder	1 set	Slide Board	2 x 30
Plyometrics #'s	17 (add sprint), 20, 24	Plyometrics #'s	12, 14, 15, 21

Day 2		Day 4	
Rotator Cuff Warm-up	x 1	Rotator Cuff Warm-up	x 1
Neck (4-Way)	1 x 10	Neck (4-Way)	1 x 10
Pull-ups	2 x 10	Incline Pull-ups	2 x 15
Stiff Leg Dead Lift	2 x 15 TS	Good Mornings	2 x 15 TS
Leg Curls (Light)	2 x 15	Leg Curls (Light)	2 x 15
Power Cleans	1 x 8, 3 x 6	Dead Lift	4 x 6
Power Shrugs	4 x 8	Power Squat	1 x 8, 3 x 5
Lunges	3 x 8	Leg Sled	1 x 8, 1 x 6, 2 x 4
Leg Curls, Single	3 x 10	Close Grip Lat Pull-downs	3 x 10
Seated Rows	3 x 8	DB One Arm Rows	3 x 8
Straight Lat Pull-downs	3 x 10	Lat Pull-downs	3 x 10
Straight Bar Curls	3 x 8	DB Hammer Curls	3 x 10
DB Curls	3 x 8	E-Z Bar Curls	3 x 10

Hip Routine			Hip Routine		
Back Stabilization			Back Stabilization		
Med Ball Routine #'s		1, 2, 6	Med Ball Routine #'s		12, 14, 15, 16

Peak/Transition Phase

Day 1		Day 3	
Rotator Cuff Warm-up	x 1	Rotator Cuff Warm-up	x 1
Supine Neck	1 x 40	Prone Neck	1 x 40
Push-ups	2 x 20	Close Grip Incline Push-Up	2 x 30
DB Lying Flys (Light)	2 x 15 SS	DB Incline Flys (Light)	2 x 15 SS
Bench Press	1 x 8, 1 x 6, 2 x 4	Close Grip Bench Press	3 x 8
Incline Press	1 x 8, 1 x 6, 2 x 3	DB Incline Press	4 x 6
Med Ball Chest Pass	4 x 10 SS	Med Ball Supine Drops	4 x 10 SS
DB Upright Rows	3 x 8	DB Front Raises	3 x 8
DB Shrugs	3 x 8 SS	DB Lateral Raises	3 x 8 SS
Dips	3 x 12	DB Tricep Extension	4 x 8
Abdominal #1		Abdominal #2	
Plyometrics #'s	6, 11, 12	Plyometrics #'s	14, 22, 23

Day 2		Day 4	
Rotator Cuff Warm-up	x 1	Rotator Cuff Warm-up	
Neck (4-Way)	1 x 10	Neck (4-Way)	1 x 10
Pull-ups	2 x 10	Incline Pull-ups	2 x 12
Good Mornings	2 x 15 TS	Good Mornings	2 x 15 TS
Torso Twists	2 x 20	Torso Twists	2 x 20
Power Cleans	1 x 6, 3 x 3	*DB Hang Clean Combo	3 x 5
Power Squat	1 x 8, 1 x 6, 1 x 4	DB One Arm Rows	3 x 8
Squat Jumps	3 x 10 SS	Lat Pull-downs	3 x 8
Leg Extensions	2 x 10	T-Bar Rows	3 x 8 SS
Leg Curls	2 x 10 SS	Back Stabilization	
Seated Rows	3 x 10	Ladder	1 set
Pull-overs	3 x 10 SS	Med Ball Routine #'s	14, 15, 16
Hip Routine			
Med Ball Routine #'s	2, 4, 6		

* DB Hang Clean Combo: Perform DB hang clean, DB push press, and DB squat for 1 repetition.

FOOTBALL/RUGBY (QUARTERBACKS)

Introduction Phase

Day 1			Day 3		
Rotator Cuff Warm-up	x 1		Rotator Cuff Warm-up	x 1	
Decline Push-ups	2 x 15		Incline Push-ups	2 x 15	
Torso Twists	2 x 20 SS		Torso Twists	2 x 20 SS	
Bench Press	3 x 15		DB Bench Press	3 x 15	
Incline Press	3 x 10		DB Incline Press	3 x 12	
DB Lying Flys	3 x 15		DB Incline Flys	3 x 10	
DB Upright Rows	3 x 15		DB Standing Military	3 x 12	
DB Shrugs	3 x 20 SS		DB Front Raises	3 x 15	
DB Reverse Lateral Raises	3 x 15		DB Lateral Raises	3 x 15 SS	
DB Tricep Extension	3 x 12		Tricep Push-down	3 x 15	
DB Tricep Kickback	3 x 12		DB Lying Tricep Extension	3 x 15	
Bench Dips	2 x 15		Dips	2 x 10	
Wrist Flexion	2 x 20		Wrist Extension	2 x 20	
Abdominal #1			Abdominal #2		

Day 2			Day 4		
Rotator Cuff Warm-up	x 1		Rotator Cuff Warm-up	x 1	
Neck (4-Way)	1 x 10		Neck (4-Way)	1 x 10	
Pull-ups	2 x 5		Incline Pull-ups	2 x 10	
Torso Twists	2 x 20 SS		Good Mornings	2 x 15 SS	
DB Hang Cleans	3 x 10		Hang Cleans	3 x 8	
DB Squat	3 x 12		Power Squat	3 x 10	
DB Step-ups	3 x 10		Lateral Lunges	3 x 10	
Leg Curls	3 x 10 SS		T-Bar Rows	3 x 12	
Seated Rows	3 x 15		Straight Bar Pull-downs	3 x 15 SS	
DB Hammer Curls	3 x 10		DB Seated Curls	3 x 10	
DB Incline Curls	3 x 15		Straight Bar Curls	3 x 15	
Hip Routine			Hip Routine		
Back Stabilization			Back Stabilization		

Strength Phase

Day 1			Day 3		
Rotator Cuff Warm-up	x 1		Rotator Cuff Warm-up	x 1	

Push-ups	2 x 15	Decline Push-ups	2 x 10
DB Lying Flys	2 x 15 SS	DB Incline Flys	2 x 15 SS
Bench Press	1 x 8, 3 x 8	DB Bench Press	3 x 8
Incline Press	3 x 8	DB Incline Press	3 x 8
Military Press	4 x 8	DB Upright Rows	3 x 10
DB Bent-over Lateral Raises	3 x 10	DB Front Raises	3 x 10
DB Bent-over Front Raises	3 x 10 SS	DB Lateral Raises	3 x 10 SS
Dips	3 x 10	Tricep Push-down	3 x 10
DB Tricep Extension	3 x 10	DB Tricep Kickback	3 x 10
Rice Routine		Rice Routine	
Ladder	2 sets	Slide Board	2 x 40
Abdominal #1		Med Ball Abdominal	

Day 2		Day 4	
Rotator Cuff Warm-up	x 1	Rotator Cuff Warm-up	x 1
Pull-ups	2 x 8	Incline Pull-ups	2 x 10
Torso Twists	2 x 20 TS	Good Mornings	2 x 15 TS
Back Extension	2 x 10	Twisting Back Extension	2 x 20
Power Cleans	3 x 8	Hang Snatch	3 x 8
Power Squat	1 x 10, 2 x 8	Hang Cleans	3 x 8
Lateral Lunges	3 x 10	Walking Lunges	3 x 10
T-Bar Rows	3 x 10	Seated Rows	3 x 10
Lat Pull-downs	3 x 10 SS	Straight Pulldowns	3 x 10 SS
DB Curls	3 x 10	DB Hammer Curls	3 x 10
Straight Bar Curls	3 x 10	DB Seated Curls	3 x 10
Standing Calves, Single	2 x 25	Seated Calves	2 x 25
Hip Routine		Hip Routine	
Back Stabilization		Back Stabilization	

Power Phase

Day 1		Day 3	
Rotator Cuff Warm-up	x 2	Rotator Cuff Warm-up	x 2
Incline Push-ups	2 x 20	Decline Push-ups	2 x 20
Torso Twists	2 x 20 SS	Torso Twists	2 x 20 SS
Bench Press	1 x 8, 3 x 6	DB Bench Press	1 x 8, 3 x 6
Incline Press	1 x 8, 1 x 4, 2 x 4	DB Incline Flys	3 x 10
Military Press	1 x 8, 3 x 6	DB Standing Military	3 x 10
Med Ball Over-head Pass	4 x 10 SS	Med Ball Prone Push	3 x 10 SS
DB Bent-over Front Raises	3 x 10	DB Bent-over Lateral Raise	3 x 10
DB Lateral Raises	3 x 10 SS	DB Upright Row	3 x 10 SS
Dips	2 x 10	Dips	2 x 10
DB Tricep Extension	3 x 8	Tricep Push-down	3 x 8

Rice Routine		Rice Routine	
Ladder	1 set	Slide Board	2 x 20
Med Ball Abdominal		Abdominal #2	
Plyometrics #'s	2, 9, 12, 13	Plyometrics #'s	14, 16, 22, 23

Day 2		Day 4	
Rotator Cuff Warm-up	x 1	Rotator Cuff Warm-up	x 1
Neck (4-Way)	1 x 10	Neck (4-Way)	1 x 10
Pull-ups	2 x 8	Incline Pull-ups	2 x 10
Good Mornings	2 x 15 SS	DB Stiff Leg Dead Lift	2 x 15 SS
Power Cleans	3 x 6	Hang Snatch	3 x 5
Leg Sled	1 x 8, 1 x 6, 2 x 4	Quarter Squat	3 x 8
Squat Jumps	4 x 10 SS	Lateral Cone Hops	3 x 10 SS
Standing Lat Pull-downs	3 x 8	Seated Rows	3 x 10
DB One Arm Rows	3 x 10 SS	DB Pull-overs	3 x 10 SS
Lateral Lunges	2 x 8	T-Bar Rows	2 x 8
Leg Extensions	2 x 10 TS	Leg Extensions	2 x 10
Leg Curls	2 x 10	Leg Curls	2 x 10 SS
DB Incline Hammer Curls	3 x 8	Straight Bar Curls	3 x 8
E-Z Bar Curls	2 x 10	DB Curls	2 x 10
Hip Routine		Back Stabilization	
Med Ball Routine #'s	5, 7, 9	Med Ball Routine #'s	13, 15, 16

Peak/Transition Phase

Day 1		Day 3	
Rotator Cuff Warm-up	x 2	Rotator Cuff Warm-up	x 2
Lying Flys (Light)	2 x 15	Incline Flys (Light)	2 x 15
Push-ups	2 x 10 SS	Incline Push-ups	2 x 10 SS
Bench Press	1 x 8, 1 x 6, 2 x 4	DB Bench Press	3 x 8
Incline Press	1 x 8, 1 x 6, 1 x 3	Military Press	1 x 8, 1 x 6, 1 x 4
Med Ball Over-head Pass	3 x 10 SS	Med Ball Supine Drops	3 x 10 SS
DB Upright Rows	3 x 10	DB Front Raises	3 x 10
DB Bent-over Lateral Raises	3 x 10 SS	DB Lateral Raises	3 x 10 SS
Dips	2 x 15	Dips	2 x 15
Ladder	1 Set	Slide Board	1 x 20
Abdominal #1		Med Ball Abdominal	
Plyometrics #'s	1, 3, 6, 9	Plyometrics #'s	12, 14, 27, 30

Day 2		Day 4	
Rotator Cuff Warm-up	x 1	Rotator Cuff Warm-up	x 1
Good Mornings	2 x 15	Good Mornings	2 x 15

Torso Twists	2 x 20 SS
Power Cleans	3 x 5
Power Squat	1 x 8, 1 x 6, 2 x 4
Double Leg Speed Hops	4 x 10 SS
Lat Pull-downs	3 x 12
DB One Arm Rows	3 x 10
Leg Extensions	2 x 10
Leg Curls	2 x 10 SS
Hip Routine	
Med Ball Routine #'s	7, 9, 10

Torso Twists	2 x 20 SS
Hang Snatch	3 x 5
Leg Sled	1 x 8, 1 x 6, 2 x 3
Single Leg Speed Hops	4 x 10 SS
Seated Rows	3 x 10
DB Pull-overs	3 x 10
Leg Extensions	2 x 10
Leg Curls	2 x 10 SS
Back Stabilization	
Med Ball Routine #'s	12, 13, 16

FOOTBALL/RUGBY (RECEIVERS, BACKS)

Introduction Phase

Day 1

Rotator Cuff Warm-up	x 1
Push-ups	2 x 15
Torso Twists	2 x 20 SS
Bench Press	3 x 15
Incline Press	4 x 12
DB Lying Flys	3 x 15
Rear Military	3 x 10
DB Upright Rows	3 x 15
DB Bent-over Front Raises	3 x 15 SS
DB Lying Tricep Extension	3 x 15
Dips	3 x 12
Wrist Flexion	2 x 20
Abdominal #1	

Day 3

Rotator Cuff Warm-up	x 1
Push-ups	2 x 15
Torso Twists	2 x 20 SS
DB Bench Press	3 x 12
DB Incline Press	3 x 12
DB Incline Flys	3 x 15
DB Standing Military	4 x 10
DB Front Raises	3 x 15
DB Lateral Raises	3 x 15 SS
Dips	2 x 15
DB Tricep Extension	3 x 12
Wrist Extension	2 x 20
Abdominal #2	

Day 2

Rotator Cuff Warm-up	x 1
Pull-ups	2 x 8
Good Mornings	2 x 10 SS
DB Hang Cleans	3 x 12
Hang Snatch	3 x 8
DB Step-ups	3 x 10
Leg Extensions	3 x 15
Leg Curls	3 x 15 SS
Seated Rows	3 x 15

Day 4

Rotator Cuff Warm-up	x 1
Incline Pull-ups	2 x 8
DB Stiff Leg Dead Lift	2 x 10 SS
Hang Cleans	4 x 10
Power Squat	3 x 10
Lunges	2 x 10
Leg Curls	2 x 20 SS
Lat Pull-downs	3 x 10
DB Pull-overs	3 x 15

Barbell Bent-over Rows	3 x 10	T-Bar Rows	3 x 10
Standing Calves	2 x 25	Seated Calves	2 x 25
Hip Routine		Hip Routine	
Back Stabilization		Back Stabilization	

Strength Phase

Day 1		Day 3	
Rotator Cuff Warm-up	x 1	Rotator Cuff Warm-up	x 1
Push-ups	1 x 15	Decline Push-ups	1 x 15
Neck (4-Way)	1 x 10	Neck (4-Way)	1 x 10
Torso Twists	1 x 20	Torso Twists	1 x 20
Bench Press	1 x 8, 3 x 6	DB Bench Press	3 x 8
Incline Press	1 x 8, 3 x 6	DB Incline Press	3 x 8
DB Standing Military	3 x 8	Rear Military	4 x 8
Upright Rows	3 x 10	DB Upright Rows	4 x 10
DB Bent-over Lateral Raises	3 x 10 SS	DB Reverse Lateral Raises	4 x 10 SS
DB Tricep Extension	4 x 8	DB Lying Tricep Extension	3 x 10
Dips	2 x 15	Dips	3 x 12 SS
Rice Routine		Rice Routine	
Med Ball Abdominal		Abdominal #2	

Day 2		Day 4	
Rotator Cuff Warm-up	x 1	Rotator Cuff Warm-up	x 1
Good Mornings	1 x 15	Good Mornings	1 x 15
Pull-ups	1 x 8	Incline Pull-ups	1 x 8
High Pulls	4 x 8	Power Cleans	3 x 8
Power Shrugs	3 x 8	Lunges	3 x 8
Power Squat	1 x 10, 3 x 8	DB Step-ups	2 x 10
DB Single Arm Rows	3 x 10	Leg Curls	2 x 15 SS
Lat Pull-downs	3 x 10	Pull-overs	3 x 10
Leg Extensions	3 x 10	Straight Lat Pull-down	3 x 10
Leg Curls	3 x 10 SS	T-Bar Rows	3 x 8 SS
Hip Routine		Hip Routine	
Back Stabilization		Back Stabilization	

Power Phase

Day 1		Day 3	
Rotator Cuff Warm-up	x 1	Rotator Cuff Warm-up	
Neck (4-Way)	1 x 10	Neck (4-Way)	1 x 10

Incline Push-ups	1 x 20	Decline Push-ups	1 x 15
Torso Twists	1 x 20	Torso Twists	1 x 20
Bench Press	1 x 8, 4 x 5	DB Bench Press	3 x 8
Incline Press	4 x 6	DB Incline Press	3 x 8
Med Ball Chest Pass	4 x 10 SS	Med Ball Over-head Pass	3 x 10 SS
DB Front Raises	3 x 10	Military Press	1 x 8, 3 x 5
DB Lateral Raises	3 x 10 TS	DB Upright Rows	3 x 8
DB Bent-over Lateral Raises	3 x 10	DB Bent-over Front Raises	3 x 10 TS
Dips	2 x 12	Rear Deltoid Pull	3 x 10
DB Tricep Extension	3 x 10	Tricep Push-down	3 x 8
Rice Routine		Bench Dips	2 x 20
Ladder	2 sets	Ladder	1 Set
Abdominal #1		Abdominal #2	
Plyometrics #'s	2, 6, 8, 9	Plyometrics #'s	11, 12, 14, 20

Day 2

Rotator Cuff Warm-up	x 1
Prone Neck Extension	2 x 30
Good Mornings	2 x 15 TS
Pull-ups	2 x 10
Power Cleans	1 x 8, 3 x 5
Leg Sled	1 x 8, 2 x 5
Step-ups	3 x 8
Leg Extensions	2 x 10
Leg Curls	2 x 12 SS
Barbell Bent-over Rows	3 x 10
Lat Pull-downs	3 x 10
Back Stabilization	
Med Ball Routine #'s	6, 7, 10, 12

Day 4

Rotator Cuff Warm-up	x 1
Supine Neck Flexion	2 x 30
Good Mornings	2 x 15 TS
Incline Pull-ups	2 x 20
*Hang Snatch Combo	3 x 5
Walking Lunges	3 x 10
Leg Curls	3 x 10 SS
Seated Rows	3 x 10
Pull-overs	3 x 8 SS
T-Bar Rows	3 x 8
Seated Calves, Single	2 x 30
Hip Routine	
Med Ball Routine #s	14, 15, 16

*Hang Snatch Combo: Perform hang snatch, power squat, and rear military press for one repetition.

Peak/Transition Phase

Day 1

Rotator Cuff Warm-up	x 1
Neck (4-Way)	1 x 10
Push-ups	2 x 20
Torso Twists	2 x 20 SS
Bench Press	1 x 8, 3 x 4
Incline Press	1 x 6, 2 x 4

Day 3

Rotator Cuff Warm-up	x 1
Neck (4-Way)	1 x 10
DB Incline Flys (Light)	2 x 15
Torso Twists	2 x 20 SS
DB Bench Press	3 x 8
DB Incline Press	3 x 6

Med Ball Supine Drops	3 x 10 SS	Med Ball Prone Push	3 x 8 SS
DB Military	3 x 8	DB Front Raises	3 x 8
DB Upright Rows	3 x 8 SS	DB Lateral Raises	3 x 8 SS
DB Tricep Extension	4 x 8	Dips	3 x 15
Med Ball Abdominal		Abdominal #2	
Ladder	1 set	Ladder	1 set
Plyometrics #s	9, 12, 14, 17 (add sprint)	Plyometrics #'s	20, 22, 23, 27

Day 2		Day 4	
Rotator Cuff Warm-up	x 1	Rotator Cuff Warm-up	x 1
Prone Neck Extension	2 x 30	Supine Neck Flexion	2 x 30
Pull-ups	2 x 10 SS	Incline Pull-ups	2 x 15 SS
Leg Extensions (Light)	1 x 20	Good Mornings	2 x 15
Leg Curls (Light)	1 x 20	Leg Curl (Light)	2 x 20 SS
Power Cleans	1 x 8, 1 x 6, 2 x 4	Hang Snatch	3 x 6
Power Squat	1 x 8, 3 x 6	Leg Sled	1 x 8, 1 x 5, 2 x 3
Double Leg Speed Hops	4 x 10 SS	Lateral Cone Hops	4 x 10 SS
Power Shrugs	3 x 8	Bent-over Barbell Rows	3 x 8
T-Bar Rows	3 x 8	Seated Rows	3 x 8
Lat Pull-downs	3 x 8	DB Pull-overs	3 x 8
Hip Routine		Back Stabilization	
Med Ball Routine #'s	10, 12, 14	Med Ball Routine #'s	9, 15, 16

FOOTBALL/RUGBY (IN SEASON PHASE)

Day 1		Day 2	
Rotator Cuff Warm-up	x 1	Rotator Cuff Warm-up	x 1
Neck (4-Way)	1 x 10	Neck (4-Way)	1 x 10
Torso Twists	3 x 20	Torso Twists	3 x 20
Push-ups	3 x 15 TS	Incline Pull-ups	3 x 10 TS
Good Mornings	3 x 15	Twisting Back Extension	3 x 20
Hang Snatch	3 x 6	DB Incline Flys	2 x 12
Quarter Squat	3 x 8	Incline Press	3 x 8
DB Pull-overs	2 x 12	Military Press	3 x 8
Lat Pull-downs	2 x 20	Upright Rows	2 x 15
Straight Bar Curls	2 x 15	Dips	2 x 15
DB Incline Hammer Curls	2 x 10	Tricep Push-down	2 x 15
Abdominal #1		Back Stabilization	
Ladder	1 set	Slide Board	1 x 20

GOLF (IN-SEASON PHASE)

Day 1		Day 2	
Rotator Cuff Warm-up	x 1	Rotator Cuff Warm-up	x 1
Decline Push-up	2 x 10	Incline Push-up	2 x 15
Twisting Back Extension	2 x 20 TS	Back Extension	2 x 20 TS
Torso Twists	2 x 10	Torso Twists	2 x 10
DB Lying Flys	2 x 15	Reverse Lunges	2 x 10
Cable Lateral Raises	2 x 15	DB Squat	2 x 15
DB Bent-over Lateral Raises	2 x 15 SS	Seated Rows	2 x 15 SS
Bench Dips	2 x 15	DB Hammer Curls	2 x 10
Rice Routine		Hip Routine	
Abdominal #1		Med Ball Abdominal	
Back Stabilization		Back Stabilization	

GOLF (OFF-SEASON PHASE)

Day 1		Day 3	
Rotator Cuff Warm-up	x 1	Rotator Cuff Warm-up	x 1
Twisting Back Extension	3 x 20	Good Mornings	3 x 20
DB Side Bends	3 x 10 TS	DB Side Bends	3 x 10 TS
Torso Twists	3 x 20	Torso Twists	3 x 20
Decline Push-ups	3 x 10	Incline Pull-ups	3 x 10
DB Lying Flys	3 x 15	Walking Lunges	3 x 10
DB Front Raises	3 x 15	DB Squat	3 x 15
DB Lateral Raises	3 x 15 TS	DB One Arm Rows	3 x 10
DB Bent-over Lateral Raises	3 x 15	DB Wrist Extension	2 x 20
Rice Routine		DB Wrist Flexion	2 x 20 SS
Abdominal #1		Abdominal #2	
Hip Routine		Hip Routine	
Back Stabilization		Back Stabilization	

Day 2	
Rotator Cuff Warm-up	x 1
Torso Twists	3 x 20
Back Extension	3 x 20 SS
Bench Dips	2 x 20
DB Hammer Curls	2 x 10

Rice Routine
Hip Routine
Med Ball Abdominal
Back Stabilization

HOCKEY/LACROSSE

Introduction Phase

Day 1	
Rotator Cuff Warm-up	x 2
Push-ups	3 x 10
Good Mornings	3 x 10 SS
Bench Press	3 x 12
Incline Press	3 x 12
DB Lying Flys	3 x 15
DB Military Press	3 x 10
DB Reverse Lateral Raises	3 x 10
Rear Deltoid Pulls	3 x 10 SS
Dips	3 x 8
DB Lying Tricep Extension	3 x 15
Rice Routine	
Abdominal #1	

Day 3	
Rotator Cuff Warm-up	x 2
Incline Push-ups	3 x 10
Twisting Back Extension	3 x 10 SS
DB Bench Press	3 x 15
DB Incline Press	3 x 15
DB Incline Flys	3 x 15
Cable Upright Rows	3 x 15
Cable Front Raises	3 x 15
Cable Lateral Raises	3 x 15
DB Hammer Curls	3 x 12
DB Incline Curls	3 x 12
Rice Routine	
Abdominal #2	

Day 2	
Rotator Cuff Warm-up	x 1
Pull-ups	3 x 5
Back Extension	3 x 10 SS
Power Squat	3 x 10
Walking Lunges	3 x 10
Leg Curls	3 x 10 SS
Straight Lat Pull-downs	3 x 15
Seated Rows	3 x 15
Seated Calves	3 x 25
Hip Routine	
Back Stabilization	

Day 4	
Rotator Cuff Warm-up	x 1
Incline Pull-ups	3 x 10
Torso Twist	3 x 10 SS
Leg Sled	3 x 15
Lateral Lunges	3 x 10
Leg Curls	3 x 10 SS
DB Pull-overs	3 x 15
DB One Arm Rows	3 x 10
Standing Calves	3 x 30
Hip Routine	
Back Stabilization	

Strength Phase

Day 1		Day 3	
Rotator Cuff Warm-up	x 2	Rotator Cuff Warm-up	x 2
Push-ups	3 x 12	Decline Push-ups	3 x 10
Good Mornings	3 x 12 SS	Twisting Back Extension	3 x 20 SS
Bench Press	3 x 8	DB Bench Press	3 x 8
Incline Press	3 x 8	DB Incline Press	3 x 8
Military Press	3 x 8	DB Upright Rows	3 x 10
Cable Lateral Raises	3 x 10	Cable Front Raises	3 x 10
DB Bent-over Lateral Raises	3 x 10 SS	DB Bent-over Front Raises	3 x 10 SS
Dips	3 x 10	DB Incline Curls	3 x 10
DB Tricep Extension	3 x 10	Straight Bar Curls	3 x 10
Abdominal #1		Med Ball Abdominal	

Day 2		Day 4	
Rotator Cuff Warm-up	x 1	Rotator Cuff Warm-up	x 1
Pull-ups	3 x 10	Incline Pull-ups	3 x 12
Back Extension	3 x 15 SS	Torso Twists	3 x 20 SS
Hang Cleans	3 x 8	Hang Snatch	3 x 8
Power Squat	3 x 8	Reverse Lunges	3 x 10
Leg Curls	3 x 10 SS	Leg Curls	3 x 10 SS
Straight Lat Pull-downs	3 x 12	DB Pull-overs	3 x 10
Seated Rows	3 x 12	T-Bar Rows	3 x 10
Seated Calves	3 x 30	Standing Calves, Single	3 x 20
Hip Routine		Hip Routine	
Back Stabilization		Back Stabilization	

Power Phase

Day 1		Day 3	
Rotator Cuff Warm-up	x 2	Rotator Cuff Warm-up	x 2
Push-ups	3 x 15	Decline Push-ups	3 x 15
Good Mornings	3 x 15 TS	Twisting Back Extension	3 x 20 TS
Torso Twists	3 x 20	Torso Twists	3 x 20
Bench Press	1 x 8, 2 x 6, 1 x 4	DB Bench Press	3 x 8
Med Ball Chest Pass	3 x 10 SS	Med Ball Over-head Pass	3 x 10 SS
Incline Press	1 x 8, 2 x 6	DB Incline Press	3 x 8
Military Press	3 x 8	DB Upright Rows	3 x 10
DB Front Raises	3 x 10	DB Bent-over Lateral Raises	3 x 10
DB Lateral Raises	3 x 10 SS	DB Bent-over Front Raises	3 x 10 SS
Dips	3 x 12	Straight Bar Curls	3 x 10

Tricep Push-down	3 x 10	DB Incline Hammer Curls	3 x 10
Abdominal #1		Med Ball Abdominal	
Ladder	2 sets	Slide Board	2 x 40
Plyometrics #'s	2, 12, 16, 21 (add sprint)	Plyometrics #'s	22, 23, 27, 30

Day 2		Day 4	
Rotator Cuff Warm-up	x 1	Rotator Cuff Warm-up	x 1
Pull-ups	3 x 10	Incline Pull-ups	3 x 15
Back Extension	3 x 15 SS	Torso Twist	3 x 20 SS
Hang Snatch	3 x 5	Power Cleans	3 x 8
Double Leg Speed Hops	3 x 10 SS	Single Leg Speed Hops	3 x 10 SS
Power Squat	1 x 8, 3 x 6	Lunges (4-Way)	3 x 5
Leg Extensions	3 x 10	Leg Extensions, Single	2 x 10
Leg Curls	3 x 10 SS	Leg Curls, Single	2 x 10 SS
Lat Pull-downs	3 x 10	DB One Arm Rows	3 x 8
Seated Rows	3 x 10	Pull-overs	3 x 8
Hip Routine		Back Stabilization	
Med Ball Routine #'s	6, 7, 9	Med Ball Routine #'s	12, 14, 16

Peak/Transition Phase

Day 1		Day 3	
Rotator Cuff Warm-up	x 2	Rotator Cuff Warm-up	x 2
Push-ups	2 x 20	Decline Push-ups	2 x 15
Good Mornings	2 x 20 SS	Twisting Back Extension	2 x 12 SS
Bench Press	1 x 8, 1 x 6, 2 x 3	DB Bench Press	3 x 8
Med Ball Chest Pass	4 x 10 SS	Med Ball Over-head Pass	3 x 10 SS
Incline Press	1 x 8, 1 x 6, 1 x 4	DB Incline Press	3 x 8
Military Press	3 x 6	DB Upright Rows	2 x 10
DB Front Raises	2 x 10	DB Bent-over Lateral Raises	2 x 10
DB Lateral Raises	2 x 10 SS	DB Bent-over Front Raises	2 x 10 SS
Dips	2 x 15	Straight Bar Curls	2 x 10
DB Lying Tricep Extension	2 x 10	DB Incline Curls	2 x 10
Abdominal #1		Med Ball Abdominal	
Ladder	1 Set	Slide Board	2 x 20
Plyometrics #'s	1, 9, 12	Plyometrics #'s	15, 20, 30

Day 2		Day 4	
Rotator Cuff Warm-up	x 1	Rotator Cuff Warm-up	x 1
Pull-ups	2 x 12	Incline Pull-ups	2 x 10
Back Extension	2 x 20 SS	Torso Twist	2 x 20 SS
Hang Snatch	3 x 5	Power Cleans	3 x 6
Lateral Cone Hops	3 x 10	Ice Skaters	3 x 10 SS

Leg Extensions	2 x 10	Lateral Lunges	2 x 10
Leg Curls	2 x 10 SS	Leg Curls	2 x 10 SS
Lat Pull-downs	2 x 10	DB One Arm Rows	2 x 8
Seated Rows	2 x 10	Pull-overs	2 x 8
Back Stabilization		Hip Routine	
Med Ball Routine #'s	6, 10, 12	Med Ball Routine #'s	13, 15, 16

HOCKEY/LACROSSE (IN-SEASON PHASE)

Day 1		Day 2	
Rotator Cuff Warm-up	x 2	Rotator Cuff Warm-up	x 1
Push-ups	2 x 10	Pull-ups	2 x 8
Good Mornings	2 x 20 TS	Extension	2 x 20 TS
Torso Twists	2 x 20	Torso Twists	2 x 20
DB Bench Press	3 x 12	Hang Snatch	3 x 10
Med Ball Chest Pass	3 x 10 SS	Lateral Cone Hops	3 x 10 SS
Incline Press	2 x 8	Leg Extensions	2 x 10
DB Military Press	3 x 8	Leg Curls	2 x 10 SS
DB Bent-over Front Raises	2 x 10	Lat Pull-downs	2 x 10
DB Bent-over Lateral Raises	2 x 10 SS	Seated Rows	2 x 10
Dips	3 x 15	Med Ball Abdominal	
Straight Bar Curls	3 x 10	Hip Routine	
Abdominal #1		Back Stabilization	

RACQUET SPORTS

Introductory Phase

Day 1		Day 3	
Rotator Cuff Warm-up	x 1	Rotator Cuff Warm-up	x 1
Push-ups	3 x 10	Decline Push-ups	3 x 10
DB Bench Press	3 x 15	DB Incline Press	3 x 15
DB Lying Flys	3 x 15	DB Incline Flys	3 x 15
DB Standing Military	3 x 12	DB Upright Rows	3 x 15
DB Bent-over Front Raises	3 x 15	DB Front Raises	3 x 15
DB Bent-over Lateral Raises	3 x 15	DB Lateral Raises	3 x 15
Bench Dips	3 x 10	DB Tricep Kickback	3 x 12
DB Tricep Extension	3 x 12	Tricep Push-down	

Rice Routine		Rice Routine	
Abdominal #1		Abdominal #2	
Back Stabilization		Back Stabilization	

Day 2		Day 4	
Rotator Cuff Warm-up	x 1	Rotator Cuff Warm-up	x 1
Pull-ups	3 x 5	Incline Pull-ups	3 x 8
Torso Twists	2 x 20	Torso Twists	2 x 20
Good Mornings	2 x 10 SS	Good Mornings	2 x 10 SS
DB Squat	3 x 20	Leg Sled	3 x 15
Walking Lunges	2 x 10	Step-ups	3 x 10
DB Stiff Leg Dead Lift	2 x 10 TS	Leg Extensions	2 x 20
Leg Curls	2 x 10	Leg Curls	2 x 20 SS
DB One Arm Rows	3 x 12	Seated Rows	3 x 12
DB Incline Curls	3 x 10	Straight Bar Curl	3 x 12
E-Z Bar Curl	3 x 10	DB Hammer Curl	3 x 10
Hip Routine		Hip Routine	

Strength Phase

Day 1		Day 3	
Rotator Cuff Warm-up	x 2	Rotator Cuff Warm-up	x 2
Push-ups	3 x 12	Decline Push-ups	3 x 12
DB Bench Press	3 x 10	DB Incline Press	3 x 10
DB Lying Flys	3 x 12	DB Incline Flys	3 x 12
DB Reverse Lateral Raises	3 x 12	Cable Front Raises	3 x 12
DB Upright Rows	3 x 12 SS	Cable Lateral Raises	3 x 12
DB Bent-over Lateral Raises	3 x 12	DB Bent-over Front Raises	3 x 12
Bench Dips	3 x 12	DB Tricep Extension	3 x 10
DB Tricep Kickback	3 x 10	Dips	2 x 5
Rice Routine		Rice Routine	
Med Ball Routine #'s	6, 7, 9	Med Ball Routine #'s	12, 13, 16
Abdominal #1		Abdominal #2	

Day 2		Day 4	
Rotator Cuff Warm-up	x 2	Rotator Cuff Warm-up	x 2
Pull-ups	3 x 5	Pull-ups	3 x 5
Torso Twists	2 x 20	Torso Twists	2 x 20
Back Extension	2 x 15 SS	Twisting Back Extension	2 x 10 SS
Power Squat	3 x 10	Leg Sled, Single	3 x 10
4-Way Lunges	2 x 10	Leg Extensions	3 x 10
Lat Pull-downs	3 x 12	Leg Curls	3 x 10 SS
Seated Rows	3 x 12	DB Pull-overs	3 x 10

DB Incline Hammer Curls	3 x 10	DB One Arm Rows	3 x 10
Hip Routine		Hip Routine	
Back Stabilization		Back Stabilization	
Ladder	1 set	Ladder	1 set

Power Phase

Day 1		Day 3	
Rotator Cuff Warm-up	x 2	Rotator Cuff Warm-up	x 2
Push-ups	3 x 15	Decline Push-ups	3 x 12
DB Bench Press	1 x 8, 3 x 6	DB Incline Press	3 x 8
DB Lying Flys	3 x 10	DB Incline Flys	3 x 10
DB Standing Military Press	3 x 8	DB Upright Rows	3 x 10
Cable Front Raises	3 x 10	DB Bent-over Front Raises	3 x 10
Cable Lateral Raises	3 x 10	DB Bent-over Lat Raises	3 x 10
Dips	3 x 10	Bench Dips	3 x 10
DB Tricep Extension	3 x 8	DB Tricep Kickback	3 x 10
Rice Routine		Rice Routine	
Back Stabilization		Back Stabilization	
Abdominal #1		Abdominal #2	
Plyometrics#'s	3, 12, 14	Plyometrics #'s	21, 22, 23

Day 2		Day 4	
Rotator Cuff Warm-up	x 2	Rotator Cuff Warm-up	x 2
Pull-ups	3 x 8	Pull-ups	3 x 8
Twisting Back Extension	3 x 10 SS	Good Mornings	3 x 15 SS
Front Squat	3 x 8	Hang Cleans	3 x 8
Leg Sled, Single	3 x 8	4-Way Lunges	1 x 10
DB Step-ups	3 x 8	Leg Extensions	3 x 10
Leg Curls	3 x 10	Leg Curls	3 x 10
Seated Rows	3 x 10	DB One Arm Rows	3 x 10
Lat Pull-down Close Grip	3 x 10	DB Pull-overs	3 x 10 SS
DB Incline Curls	3 x 10	Straight Bar Curls	3 x 10
DB Hammer Curls	3 x 10	DB Curls	3 x 10
Hip Routine		Hip Routine	
Ladder	2 sets	Ladder	2 sets
Med Ball Routine #'s	2, 5, 10	Med Ball Routine #'s	13, 15, 16

Peak/Transition Phase

Day 1		Day 3	
Rotator Cuff Warm-up	x 2	Rotator Cuff Warm-up	x 2
Push-up	2 x 20	Decline Push-ups	2 x 15
DB Bench Press	1 x 8, 1 x 6, 2 x 4	DB Incline Press	1 x 8, 3 x 6
DB Lying Flys	3 x 10	DB Incline Flys	3 x 10
Upright Rows	3 x 8	DB Front Raises	3 x 10
DB Bent-over Front Raises	3 x 10	DB Lateral Raises	3 x 10
DB Bent-over Lateral Raises	3 x 10	Rear Deltoid Pulls	3 x 10
Dips	2 x 10	Bench Dips	2 x 20
DB Tricep Extension	2 x 10	Tricep Push-down	2 x 10
Rice Routine		Rice Routine	
Med Ball Routine		Med Ball Routine	
Abdominal #1		Abdominal #2	
Back Stabilization		Back Stabilization	
Plyometrics #'s	15, 17, 30	Plyometrics #'s	16, 28, 29

Day 2		Day 4	
Rotator Cuff Warm-up	x 2	Rotator Cuff Warm-up	x 2
Pull-ups	2 x 10	Pull-ups	2 x 10
Twisting Back Extension	2 x 10 SS	Good Mornings	2 x 10 SS
Power Squat	1 x 8, 3 x 6	Hang Cleans	4 x 6
4-Way Lunges	1 x 10	Leg Sled, Single	3 x 8
Leg Extensions	2 x 10	Leg Extensions, Single	2 x 10
Leg Curls	2 x 10	Leg Curls, Single	2 x 10
Seated Rows	2 x 10	Lat Pull-downs	2 x 10
DB Pull-overs	2 x 10 SS	Straight Bar Pull-downs	2 x 10
DB Incline Hammer Curls	2 x 10	DB Curls	2 x 10
Straight Bar Curls	2 x 10	E-Z Bar Curls	2 x 10
Hip Routine		Hip Routine	
Ladder	1 set	Ladder	1 set

RACQUET SPORTS (IN-SEASON PHASE)

Day 1		Day 2	
Rotator Cuff Warm-up	x 2	Rotator Cuff Warm-up	x 2
Push-ups	1 x 10	Decline Push-ups	1 x 10
Incline Pull-ups	1 x 5	Dips	1 x 8
DB Bench Press	2 x 15	DB Incline Press	3 x 8
DB Lying Flys	2 x 10 SS	DB Incline Flys	3 x 10 SS

DB Military Press	2 x 8
DB Upright Rows	2 x 12
DB Front Raises	2 x 15
DB Lateral Raises	2 x 15 SS
Lateral Lunges	2 x 10
Leg Extensions	1 x 15
Leg Curls	1 x 15
Med Ball Abdominal	
Hip Routine	

DB Bent-over Front Raises	2 x 15
DB Bent-over Lateral Raises	2 x 15 SS
DB Squat	2 x 15
Lunges	1 x 10
Leg Curls	1 x 20
Seated Rows	3 x 15
DB Incline Hammer Curls	2 x 10
Ladder	1 Set
Back Stabilization	

RECREATION SPORTS

Beginner

Day 1

Rotator Cuff Warm-up	x 1
Push-ups	3 x 5
Torso Twists	3 x 20 SS
Bench Press	3 x 15
DB Incline Press	3 x 15
DB Incline Flys	3 x 15
DB Front Raises	3 x 15
DB Lateral Raises	3 x 15 TS
DB Bent-over Lateral Raises	3 x 15
Back Stabilization	
Abdominal #1	

Day 2

Rotator Cuff Warm-up	x 2
Back Extension	2 x 10
Straight Bar Curls	3 x 15
DB Hammer Curls	3 x 10
Tricep Push-down	3 x 15
DB Lying Tricep Extension	3 x 15
Abdominal #2	
Hip Routine	
Back Stabilization	

Day 3

Rotator Cuff Warm-up	x 1
Assisted Pull-ups	3 x 5
Torso Twists	3 x 20 SS
DB Squat	3 x 15
DB Lunges	3 x 10
Leg Extensions	3 x 15
Leg Curls	3 x 15 SS
Seated Rows	3 x 15
Lat Pull-downs	3 x 15
Abdominal #1	

Novice

Day 1		Day 3	
Rotator Cuff Warm-up	x 1	Rotator Cuff Warm-up	x 1
Push-ups	3 x 10	Incline Pull-ups	3 x 10
Torso Twists	3 x 20 SS	Torso Twists	3 x 20 SS
Bench Press	1 x 10, 3 x 8	Power Squat	1 x 10, 3 x 8
Incline Press	3 x 8	Step-ups	3 x 10
DB Incline Flys	3 x 10	Leg Extensions	3 x 10
DB Military Press	3 x 10	Leg Curls	3 x 10 SS
DB Upright Rows	3 x 10	Pull-overs	3 x 10
DB Reverse Lateral Raises	3 x 15 TS	T-Bar Rows	3 x 10
DB Bent-over Lateral Raises	3 x 15	DB One Arm Rows	3 x 10
Abdominal #1		Abdominal #1	
Back Stabilization		Back Stabilization	

Day 2	
Rotator Cuff Warm-up	x 2
Back Extension	2 x 15
Straight Bar Curls	3 x 10
DB Hammer Curls	3 x 10
DB Incline Curls	3 x 10
DB Tricep Extension	3 x 10
DB Lying Tricep Extension	3 x 10
DB Tricep Kickback	3 x 10
Med Ball Abdominal	
Hip Routine	
Back Stabilization	

Advanced

Day 1		Day 3	
Rotator Cuff Warm-up	x 1	Rotator Cuff Warm-up	x 1
Torso Twists	3 x 20	Torso Twists	3 x 20
Decline Push-ups	3 x 15 SS	Pull-ups	3 x 10 SS
Bench Press	1 x 8, 3 x 6	Hang Cleans	3 x 8
Incline Press	4 x 6	Power Squat	1 x 8, 3 x 6
DB Incline Flys	3 x 8	Walking Lunges	3 x 10
Military Press	3 x 8	Leg Curls	3 x 10 SS
Upright Rows	3 x 10	Straight Lat Pull-downs	3 x 10
Cable Front Raises	3 x 10	Pull-overs	3 x 8
Rear Deltoid Pulls	3 x 10	T-Bar Rows	3 x 8 SS

Abdominal #1
Back Stabilization

Abdominal #2
Back Stabilization

Day 2
Rotator Cuff Warm-up	x 2
Twisting Back Extension	3 x 20
Dips	3 x 15
Straight Bar Curl	3 x 8
DB Incline Hammer Curls	3 x 8
DB Seated Curls	3 x 10
DB Tricep Extension	4 x 8
DB Lying Tricep Extension	3 x 10
Med Ball Abdominal	
Hip Routine	
Back Stabilization	

SOCCER

Introduction Phase

Day 1
Rotator Cuff Warm-up	x 1
Neck (Four-way)	1 x 10
Push-ups	2 x 10
Torso Twists	2 x 20 SS
DB Bench Press	3 x 15
DB Lying Flys	3 x 15
DB Standing Military Press	3 x 10
DB Upright Rows	3 x 12
DB Bent-over Front Raises	3 x 10
Bench Dips	2 x 10
Tricep Push-down	3 x 15
Abdominal #1	

Day 2
Torso Twists	2 x 20
Twisting Back Extension	2 x 10 SS
High Pulls	3 x 10
Hang Cleans	2 x 10
DB Step-ups	3 x 10

Day 3
Rotator Cuff Warm-up	x 1
Neck (Four-way)	1 x 10
Incline Push-ups	2 x 10
Torso Twists	2 x 20 SS
DB Incline Press	3 x 15
DB Incline Flys	3 x 15
DB Front Raises	3 x 15
DB Lateral Raises	3 x 15 TS
DB Bent-over Lateral Raises	3 x 15
DB Hammer Curls	3 x 10
Straight Bar Curls	2 x 15
Abdominal #2	

Day 4
Good Mornings	2 x 15
Pull-ups	2 x 5 SS
DB Squat	3 x 15
DB Walking Lunges	2 x 10
Leg Extensions	2 x 20

Leg Curls	2 x 15 SS	Leg Curls	2 x 20 SS
Seated Rows	3 x 15	DB Pull-overs	3 x 15
Lat Pull-downs	3 x 15	Straight Bar Pull-downs	3 x 15
Hip Routine		Hip Routine	
Back Stabilization		Back Stabilization	

Strength Phase

Day 1

Rotator Cuff Warm-up	x 1
Prone Neck Extension	2 x 20
Push-ups	2 x 12
Torso Twists	2 x 20 SS
DB Bench Press	3 x 10
DB Lying Flys	3 x 12
DB Seated Military Press	3 x 10
Upright Rows	3 x 10
DB Bent-over Front Raises	3 x 10 SS
Bench Dips	2 x 12
DB Lying Tricep Extension	3 x 12
Abdominal #1	

Day 3

Rotator Cuff Warm-up	x 1
Supine Neck Flexion	2 x 20
Incline Push-ups	2 x 15
Torso Twists	2 x 20 SS
DB Incline Press	3 x 10
DB Incline Flys	3 x 12
DB Front Raises	3 x 12
DB Lateral Raises	3 x 12 TS
Rear Deltoid Pulls	3 x 12
DB Incline Hammer Curls	3 x 10
Straight Bar Curls	2 x 12
Med Ball Abdominal	

Day 2

Torso Twists	2 x 20
Twisting Back Extension	2 x 20 SS
High Pulls	2 x 8
Hang Cleans	3 x 8
DB Step-ups	2 x 10
Leg Curls	2 x 10 SS
Seated Rows	3 x 12
Lat Pull-downs	2 x 10
Hip Routine	
Back Stabilization	

Day 4

Good Mornings	2 x 15
Incline Pull-ups	2 x 8
Power Squat	3 x 10
Lateral Lunges	2 x 10
Leg Extensions	2 x 15
Leg Curls	2 x 15 SS
DB Pull-overs	3 x 12
Straight Bar Pull-downs	2 x 10
Hip Routine	
Back Stabilization	

Power Phase

Day 1

Rotator Cuff Warm-up	x 1
Prone Neck Extension	2 x 20
Push-ups	2 x 15
Torso Twists	2 x 20 SS

Day 3

Rotator Cuff Warm-up	
Supine Neck Flexion	2 x 20
Incline Push-ups	3 x 12
Torso Twists	2 x 20 SS

DB Bench Press	1 x 8, 2 x 6	DB Incline Press	1 x 10, 2 x 8
DB Lying Flys	3 x 10	DB Incline Flys	3 x 10
DB Standing Military Press	3 x 10	DB Front Raises	3 x 10
DB Bent-over Lateral Raises	3 x 10	DB Lateral Raises	3 x 10
DB Bent-over Front Raises	3 x 10 SS	Rear Deltoid Pulls	3 x 10
Dips	2 x 10	DB Hammer Curl	3 x 10
Tricep Push-down	3 x 10	Straight Bar Curl	2 x 10
Med Ball Abdominal		Abdominal #2	
Plyometrics #'s	1, 6, 7, 9	Plyometrics #'s	12, 14, 16, 18

Day 2		Day 4	
Torso Twists	2 x 20	Good Mornings	2 x 15
Twisting Back Extension	2 x 20 SS	Incline Pull-ups	2 x 10
Hang Snatch	2 x 8	Power Squat	3 x 10
Lateral Cone Hops	2 x 10 SS	Jump Squats	3 x 10 SS
Power Cleans	1 x 8, 2 x 6	Reverse Lunges	2 x 10
DB Lateral Step-ups	2 x 10	Leg Extension	3 x 10
Leg Curl	2 x 10 SS	Leg Curl	3 x 10 SS
Seated Row	3 x 10	DB Pull-over	3 x 10
Lat Pull-down	3 x 10	Straight Bar Pull-down	3 x 10
Hip Routine		Hip Routine	
Back Stabilization		Back Stabilization	

Peak/Transition Phase

Day 1		Day 3	
Rotator Cuff Warm-up	x 1	Rotator Cuff Warm-up	x 1
Torso Twists	1 x 20	Torso Twists	2 x 20
Push-ups	1 x 20	Incline Push-ups	2 x 15 SS
DB Bench Press	1 x 6, 2 x 4	DB Incline Press	1 x 8, 2 x 6
DB Lying Flys	3 x 10	DB Incline Flys	3 x 10
DB Standing Military Press	2 x 10	DB Front Raises	2 x 10
Upright Rows	2 x 10	DB Lateral Raises	2 x 10
DB Bent-over Front Raises	2 x 10	Deltoid Pulls	2 x 10
Dips	2 x 10	DB Hammer Curls	2 x 10
DB Tricep Extension	3 x 10	Straight Bar Curls	2 x 10
Med Ball Abdominal		Abdominal #2	
Plyometrics #'s	20, 21, 22, 23	Plyometrics#'s	5, 12 26, 27

Day 2		Day 4	
Torso Twists	1 x 20	Good Mornings	1 x 15
Neck (4-way)	1 x 10	Neck (4-way)	1 x 10

Twisting Back Extension	1 x 20	Pull-ups	1 x 8
Hang Snatch	2 x 8	Power Squat	3 x 8
Single 6-Inch Box Jumps	2 x 10 SS	Lateral Box Jumps	3 x 10 SS
Power Cleans	1 x 6, 2 x 4	Walking Lunges	2 x 10
DB Lateral Step-ups	2 x 10	Leg Extensions	2 x 10
Leg Curls	2 x 10 SS	Leg Curls	2 x 10 SS
Seated Rows	2 x 10	DB One Arm Rows	2 x 10
Lat Pull-downs	2 x 10	Straight Bar Pull-downs	2 x 10
Hip Routine		Back Stabilization	

SOCCER (IN-SEASON PHASE)

Day 1

Rotator Cuff Warm-up	x 1	
Prone Neck Extension	1 x 20	
Twisting Back Extension	1 x 20	
Push-ups	2 x 15	
DB Lying Flys	2 x 15	SS
Hang Cleans	2 x 8	
Box Jumps	2 x 20	SS
DB Walking Lunges	2 x 10	
Leg Curls	2 x 10	SS
DB Upright Rows	2 x 10	
DB Bent-over Front Raises	2 x 10	SS
Seated Rows	2 x 10	
Bench Dips	1 x 20	
Abdominal #1		

Day 2

Rotator Cuff Warm-up	x 1	
Supine Neck Flexion	1 x 20	
Torso Twists	2 x 20	
Incline Pull-ups	2 x 10	
DB Incline Flys	2 x 15 SS	
DB Squat	2 x 10	
Squat Jump	2 x 10 SS	
Leg Extensions	2 x 15	
Leg Curls	2 x 10	
DB Front Raises	2 x 15	
DB Bent-over Lateral Raises	2 x 15 SS	
Lat Pull-downs	2 x 12	
DB Hammer Curls	2 x 10	
Back Stabilization		

SWIMMING/WATER POLO

Introduction Phase

Day 1

Rotator Cuff Warm-up	x 2
Torso Twists	1 x 20
Incline Push-up	3 x 10

Day 3

Rotator Cuff Warm-up	x 2
Torso Twists	1 x 20
Decline Push-ups	3 x 10

DB Lying Flys	3 x 15 SS		DB Incline Flys	3 x 15 SS
DB Bench Press	3 x 15		DB Incline Press	3 x 15
DB Standing Military	3 x 15		DB Bent-over Front Raises	3 x 15
DB Upright Rows	3 x 15		DB Lateral Raises	3 x 15 TS
DB Bent-over Lateral Raises	3 x 15 SS		DB Front Raises	3 x 15
Bench Dips	2 x 15		DB Lying Tricep Extension	3 x 15
DB Tricep Extension	3 x 15		DB Tricep Kickback	3 x 15
Abdominal #1			Abdominal #2	

Day 2			Day 4	
Rotator Cuff Warm-up	x 2		Rotator Cuff Warm-up	x 2
Pull-ups	2 x 5		Incline Pull-ups	2 x 8
Back Extension	2 x 10 SS		Twisting Back Extension	2 x 10 SS
Walking Lunges	2 x 10		DB Squat	3 x 20
DB Stiff Leg Dead Lift	2 x 10 TS		Leg Extension	3 x 15
Leg Curls	2 x 10		Leg Curls	3 x 15 SS
Straight Bar Pull-downs	3 x 20		Lat Pull-downs	3 x 20
DB Pull-overs	3 x 15		Seated Rows	3 x 15
DB Hammer Curls	3 x 10		DB Curls	3 x 10
DB Incline Curls	2 x 10		Straight Bar Curls	2 x 15
Reverse Back Extension	2 x 10		Reverse Back Extension	2 x 10
Hip Routine			Hip Routine	
Back Stabilization			Back Stabilization	

Strength Phase

Day 1			Day 3	
Rotator Cuff Warm-up	x 2		Rotator Cuff Warm-up	x 2
Torso Twists	2 x 20		Torso Twists	2 x 20
Incline Push-ups	3 x 12		Decline Push-ups	3 x 12
DB Lying Flys	3 x 12 SS		DB Incline Flys	3 x 12 SS
DB Bench Press	3 x 10		DB Incline Press	3 x 10
DB Standing Military	3 x 10		DB Bent-over Front Raises	3 x 12
Rear Deltoid Pulls	3 x 12		DB Shrugs	3 x 12 TS
DB Bent-over Lateral Raises	3 x 15 SS		DB Upright Rows	3 x 12
Dips	2 x 10		DB Lying Tricep Extension	3 x 12
Tricep Push-down	3 x 12		DB Tricep Kickback	3 x 12
Abdominal #1			Med Ball Abdominal	

Day 2			Day 4	
Rotator Cuff Warm-up	x 2		Rotator Cuff Warm-up	x 2
Pull-ups	2 x 8		Incline Pull-ups	2 x 10
Back Extension	2 x 15 SS		Twisting Back Extension	2 x 20 SS

Hang Snatch	3 x 8	Hang Clean	3 x 8
Lateral Lunges	2 x 10	Squat	3 x 8
Leg Curls	2 x 10 SS	Leg Curls	3 x 15 SS
Straight Bar Pull-downs	3 x 15	Lat Pull-downs	3 x 15
DB Pull-overs	3 x 12	T-Bar Rows	3 x 10
DB Hammer Curls	3 x 10	DB Curls	3 x 10
DB Incline Curls	2 x 10	Straight Bar Curls	2 x 15
Reverse Back Extension	2 x 15	Reverse Back Extension	2 x 15
Hip Routine		Hip Routine	
Back Stabilization		Back Stabilization	

Power Phase

Day 1		**Day 3**	
Rotator Cuff Warm-up	x 2	Rotator Cuff Warm-up	x 2
Torso Twists	2 x 20	Torso Twists	2 x 20
Med Ball Push-ups	3 x 10	Med Ball Supine Drops	3 x 10
DB Lying Flys	3 x 10 SS	DB Incline Flys	3 x 12 SS
DB Bench Press	3 x 8	DB Incline Press	3 x 10
Med Ball Over-head Pass	3 x 10 SS	Med Ball One Arm Toss	3 x 10 SS
DB Standing Military	2 x 10	DB Bent-over Front Raise	2 x 10
Upright Rows	2 x 10	DB Shrug	2 x 10
DB Bent-over Lateral Raises	2 x 10	DB Lateral Raises	2 x 10
Dips	2 x 12	DB Lying Tricep Extension	3 x 10
Tricep Push-down	3 x 10	DB Tricep Kickback	3 x 10
Abdominal #1		Med Ball Abdominal	
Plyometrics #'s	5, 11, 14	Plyometrics #'s	4, 7, 13
Day 2		**Day 4**	
Rotator Cuff Warm-up	x 2	Rotator Cuff Warm-up	x 2
Pull-ups	2 x 10	Incline Pull-ups	2 x 15
Back Extension	2 x 20 SS	Twisting Back Extension	2 x 20 SS
Hang Snatch	3 x 6	*Hang Clean Combo	3 x 5
Lateral Lunges	2 x 10	Leg Extensions	2 x 10
Leg Curls	2 x 10 SS	Leg Curls	2 x 10 SS
Straight Bar Pull-downs	3 x 15	Lat Pull-downs	3 x 15
DB Pull-overs	3 x 12	T-Bar Rows	3 x 10
DB Hammer Curls	3 x 10	DB Curls	3 x 10
DB Incline Curls	2 x 10	Straight Bar Curls	2 x 15
Reverse Back Extension	2 x 20	Reverse Back Extension	2 x 20
Hip Routine		Hip Routine	
Back Stabilization		Back Stabilization	
Med Ball Routine #'s	12, 16	Med Ball Routine #'s	5, 11

*Hang Clean Combo: Perform hang clean, front squat, and push press for 1 repetition.

Peak/Transition Phase

Day 1
Rotator Cuff Warm-up	x 2
UE Step-ups	1 x 10
Med Ball Push-ups	1 x 10
DB Lying Flys	1 x 10
DB Bench Press	1 x 8, 1 x 6, 2 x 4
Med Ball Over-head Pass	4 x 10 SS
DB Standing Military Press	3 x 8
DB Upright Rows	3 x 8
Dips	2 x 10
Abdominal #1	
Plyometrics #'s	5, 7, 32

Day 2
Rotator Cuff Warm-up	x 1
Torso Twists	2 x 20
Twisting Back Extension	2 x 20 SS
Hang Snatch	2 x 8
Box Jumps	2 x 10 SS
Straight Lat Pull-downs	2 x 10
Seated Rows	3 x 8
DB Incline Hammer Curls	2 x 10
Back Stabilization	
Med Ball Routine #'s	12, 16

Day 3
Rotator Cuff Warm-up	x 2
Decline Push-ups	1 x 15
Med Ball Walk Overs	1 x 10
DB Incline Flys	1 x 10
DB Incline Press	1 x 8, 3 x 6
Med Ball Single Toss	4 x 10 SS
Cable Lateral Raises	3 x 10
Rear Deltoid Pulls	3 x 10 SS
Bench Dips	2 x 20
Med Ball Abdominal	
Plyometrics #'s	11, 14, 18

Day 4
Rotator Cuff Warm-up	x 1
Torso Twists	2 x 20
Good Mornings	2 x 15 SS
Squat	2 x 8
Squat Jumps	2 x 10 SS
Pull-overs	2 x 10
T-Bar Rows	3 x 8
Straight Bar Curls	2 x 10
Back Stabilization	
Med Ball Routine #'s	5, 9

SWIMMING/WATER POLO (IN-SEASON PHASE)

Day 1
Rotator Cuff Warm-up	x 1
Decline Push-ups	2 x 10
Med Ball Prone Push	2 x 10 SS
DB Lying Flys	2 x 15
DB Military Press	3 x 8
DB Bent-over Lateral Raises	3 x 10
Dips	2 x 10
Abdominal #1	
Back Stabilization	

Day 2
Rotator Cuff Warm-up	x 1
Incline Pull-ups	2 x 10
Med Ball Walk Overs	2 x 10 SS
Twisting Back Extension	2 x 20
Hang Snatch	2 x 8
Squat Jumps	2 x 10 SS
DB Incline Hammer Curls	2 x 10
Med Ball Abdominal	
Hip Routine	

TRACK AND FIELD (JUMPERS)

Introduction Phase

Day 1

Rotator Cuff Warm-up	x 1
Torso Twists	2 x 20
Push-ups	2 x 10 SS
DB Bench Press	3 x 15
DB Lying Flys	3 x 15
DB Front Raises	3 x 15
DB Lateral Raises	3 x 15
Rear Deltoid Pulls	3 x 15
Bench Dips	3 x 10
Abdominal #1	

Day 3

Rotator Cuff Warm-up	x 1
Torso Twists	2 x 20
Decline Push-ups	2 x 10 SS
DB Incline Press	3 x 15
DB Incline Flys	3 x 15
DB Upright Rows	3 x 15
DB Military Press	3 x 10
DB Hammer Curls	3 x 10
Straight Bar Curls	3 x 15
Abdominal #2	

Day 2

Rotator Cuff Warm-up	x 1
Pull-ups	2 x 5
Twisting Back Extension	2 x 20 SS
High Pulls	3 x 10
Hang Cleans	3 x 10
Power Squat	3 x 10
Leg Extensions	2 x 15
Leg Curls	2 x 15 SS
Seated Rows	3 x 15
Hip Routine	
Back Stabilization	

Day 4

Rotator Cuff Warm-up	x 1
Incline Pull-ups	2 x 8
Reverse Back Extension	2 x 15 SS
DB Hang Cleans	3 x 15
DB Squat	2 x 15
DB Step-ups	3 x 10
Leg Curls	3 x 15 SS
Standing Calves	3 x 25
Straight Lat Pull-down	3 x 15
Hip Routine	
Back Stabilization	

Strength Phase

Day 1

Rotator Cuff Warm-up	
Torso Twists	2 x 20
Push-ups	2 x 15 SS
DB Bench Press	3 x 10
DB Lying Flys	3 x 12
Cable Front Raises	3 x 12
Cable Lateral Raise	3 x 12 SS
Rear Deltoid Pulls	3 x 12

Day 3

Rotator Cuff Warm-up	
Torso Twists	2 x 20
Decline Push-ups	2 x 12 SS
DB Incline Press	3 x 10
DB Incline Flys	3 x 12
Military Press	3 x 10
DB Bent-over Lateral Raises	3 x 10
Upright Rows	3 x 12 SS

DB Incline Curls	3 x 10	DB Hammer Curls	3 x 10
DB Tricep Kickback	3 x 12	Dips	3 x 12
Abdominal #1		Abdominal #2	

Day 2		Day 4	
Rotator Cuff Warm-up	x 1	Rotator Cuff Warm-up	x 1
Pull-ups	2 x 8	Incline Pull-ups	2 x 10
DB Stiff Leg Dead Lift	2 x 15 SS	Reverse Back Extension	2 x 15 SS
High Pulls	2 x 8	*DB Hang Clean Combo	3 x 5
Hang Cleans	3 x 8	Leg Extensions	2 x 10
Power Squat	3 x 8	Leg Curls	2 x 10 SS
Leg Curls	2 x 15	Straight Lat Pull-downs	3 x 10
Lat Pull-downs	3 x 10	Pull-overs	3 x 10
T-Bar Rows	3 x 12	Standing Calves, Single	3 x 20
Hip Routine		Hip Routine	
Back Stabilization		Back Stabilization	

*DB Hang Clean Combo: Perform DB hang clean, DB front squat, and DB push press for one repetition.

Power Phase

Day 1		Day 3	
Rotator Cuff Warm-up	x 1	Rotator Cuff Warm-up	x 1
Torso Twists	2 x 20	Torso Twists	2 x 20
Push-ups	2 x 20 SS	Decline Push-ups	2 x 15 SS
DB Bench Press	3 x 8	DB Incline Press	3 x 8
DB Lying Flys	3 x 10	DB Incline Flys	3 x 10
DB Front Raises	3 x 10	DB Upright Row	3 x 10
DB Lateral Raises	3 x 10	DB Military Press	3 x 8
Rear Deltoid Pulls	3 x 10	DB Reverse Lateral Raise	3 x 10
E-Z Bar Curls	3 x 10	DB Seated Curls	3 x 10
DB Tricep Extension	3 x 10	Dips	3 x 12
Abdominal #1		Med Ball Abdominal	
Plyometrics#'s	1, 5, 7, 8	Plyometrics #'s	11, 18, 29, 32

Day 2		Day 4	
Rotator Cuff Warm-up	x 1	Rotator Cuff Warm-up	x 1
Pull-ups	2 x 10	Incline Pull-ups	2 x 12
DB Stiff Leg Dead Lift	2 x 15 SS	Reverse Back Extension	2 x 15 SS
Power Cleans	1 x 8, 3 x 6	Hang Cleans	3 x 8
Single Leg Speed Hops	4 x 10 SS	Squat Jumps	3 x 10 SS
Squat	1 x 8, 2 x 6	Hang Snatch	2 x 8
Walking Lunges	3 x 10	Leg Extensions	3 x 10

Leg Curls	3 x 10 SS	Leg Curls	3 x 10 SS
Standing Calves, Single	3 x 20	Seated Calves	3 x 30
Seated Rows	3 x 10	Lat Pull-downs	3 x 10
Hip Routine		Hip Routine	
Back Stabilization		Back Stabilization	

Peak/Transition Phase

Day 1		Day 3	
Rotator Cuff Warm-up	x 1	Rotator Cuff Warm-up	x 1
Torso Twists	2 x 20	Torso Twists	2 x 20
Push-ups	2 x 10 SS	Decline Push-ups	2 x 10 SS
DB Bench Press	1 x 8, 2 x 6	DB Incline Press	1 x 8, 2 x 6
DB Lying Flys	3 x 10	DB Incline Flys	3 x 10
DB Front Raises	2 x 10	Military Press	2 x 8
DB Lateral Raises	2 x 10 TS	Upright Row	2 x 10
Rear Deltoid Pulls	2 x 10	DB Bent-over Front Raise	2 x 10
Straight Bar Curls	3 x 10	DB Seated Curls	3 x 10
DB Lying Tricep Extension	3 x 10	Bench Dips	3 x 15
Med Ball Abdominal		Abdominal #2	
Plyometrics #'s	2, 5, 10	Plyometrics #'s	18, 25, 27

Day 2		Day 4	
Rotator Cuff Warm-up	x 1	Rotator Cuff Warm-up	x 1
Pull-ups	2 x 10	Incline Pull-ups	2 x 15
Good Mornings	2 x 20 SS	Reverse Back Extension	2 x 20 SS
Power Cleans	1 x 8, 1 x 6, 1 x 4	Hang Cleans	3 x 5
Squats	3 x 8	Single Box Jumps	3 x 10 SS
Squat Jumps	3 x 10 SS	Leg Extensions, Single	3 x 10
Seated Rows	3 x 10	Leg Curls, Single	3 x 10 SS
Standing Calves, Single	2 x 30	DB One Arm Rows	3 x 10
Hip Routine		Back Stabilization	

TRACK AND FIELD (JUMPERS) (IN-SEASON PHASE)

Day 1		Day 2	
Rotator Cuff Warm-up	x 1	Rotator Cuff Warm-up	x 1
Push-ups	2 x 15	Pull-ups	2 x 8
Reverse Back Extension	2 x 15 SS	Twisting Back Extension	2 x 20
DB Bench Press	3 x 10	Power Cleans	3 x 8

DB Incline Flys	2 x 15	Squat	3 x 8
DB Front Raises	2 x 15	Squat Jumps	3 x 10 SS
DB Lateral Raises	2 x 15 SS	Leg Extensions	2 x 15
Deltoid Pulls	2 x 15	Leg Curls	2 x 15 SS
DB Lying Tricep Extension	3 x 10	Seated Calves	2 x 25
Abdominal #1		Lat Pull-downs	3 x 15
Back Stabilization		Hip Routine	

TRACK AND FIELD (POLE VAULTERS)

Introductory Phase

Day 1

Rotator Cuff Warm-up	x 2
Decline Push-ups	3 x 10
Reverse Back Extension	3 x 10 SS
DB Bench Press	3 x 15
DB Incline Flys	3 x 15
Military Press	3 x 12
Upright Rows	3 x 15
DB Reverse Lateral Raises	3 x 15
DB Tricep Extension	3 x 12
DB Lying Tricep Extension	3 x 15
DB Incline Curls	3 x 10
Abdominal #1	

Day 2

Rotator Cuff Warm-up	x 2
Pull-ups	3 x 5
Twisting Back Extension	3 x 10 SS
High Pulls	3 x 10
Hang Snatch	3 x 8
Power Squat	3 x 12
Leg Curls	3 x 15 SS
Seated Calves	3 x 25
Pull-overs	3 x 15
Hip Routine	
Back Stabilization	

Day 3

Rotator Cuff Warm-up	x 2
Push-ups	3 x 15
Back Extension	3 x 10 SS
DB Incline Press	3 x 15
DB Lying Flys	3 x 15
DB Front Raises	3 x 15
DB Bent-over Front Raises	3 x 15
DB Bent-over Lateral Raises	3 x 15 SS
Bench Dips	3 x 10
Straight Bar Curls	3 x 15
DB Hammer Curls	3 x 10
Med Ball Abdominal	

Day 4

Rotator Cuff Warm-up	x 2
Incline Pull-ups	3 x 10
Good Mornings	3 x 10 SS
Hang Cleans	3 x 10
DB Walking Lunges	3 x 10
Leg Extensions	3 x 15
Leg Curls	3 x 15 SS
Standing Calves, Single	3 x 20
Straight Lat Pull-downs	3 x 20
Hip Routine	
Back Stabilization	

Strength Phase

Day 1	
Rotator Cuff Warm-up	x 2
Decline Push-ups	3 x 12
Reverse Back Extension	3 x 12 SS
DB Bench Press	3 x 10
DB Incline Flys	3 x 10
DB Military Press	3 x 10
DB Upright Rows	3 x 12
DB Reverse Lateral Raises	3 x 12 SS
Dips	3 x 10
DB Incline Curls	3 x 10
Rice Routine	
Abdominal #1	

Day 3	
Rotator Cuff Warm-up	x 2
Push-ups	3 x 15
Back Extension	3 x 15 SS
DB Incline Press	3 x 10
DB Lying Flys	3 x 12
Cable Front Raises	3 x 12
Cable Lateral Raises	3 x 12
DB Bent-over Lateral Raises	3 x 12 SS
Bench Dips	3 x 12
DB Hammer Curls	3 x 8
Rice Routine	
Med Ball Abdominal	

Day 2	
Rotator Cuff Warm-up	x 2
Pull-ups	3 x 8
Twisting Back Extension	3 x 20 SS
High Pulls	2 x 8
Power Snatch	3 x 8
Front Squat	3 x 8
Seated Calves	3 x 25
Lat Pull-downs	3 x 12
Pull-overs	3 x 12
Hip Routine	
Back Stabilization	

Day 4	
Rotator Cuff Warm-up	x 2
Pull-ups	3 x 8
Good Mornings	3 x 15 SS
DB Hang Clean	3 x 10
DB Stiff Leg Dead Lift	3 x 10 SS
Leg Extensions	3 x 12
Leg Curls	3 x 12 SS
Standing Calves, Single	3 x 20
Straight Lat Pull-downs	3 x 15
Hip Routine	
Back Stabilization	

Power Phase

Day 1	
Rotator Cuff Warm-up	x 2
Decline Push-ups	3 x 15
Reverse Back Extension	3 x 15 SS
DB Bench Press	1 x 8, 3 x 6
DB Incline Flys	3 x 10
DB Military Press	1 x 8, 2 x 6
DB Upright Rows	3 x 10
Rear Deltoid Pulls	3 x 10 SS
Dips	3 x 12

Day 3	
Rotator Cuff Warm-up	x 2
Push-ups	3 x 20
Back Extension	3 x 20 SS
DB Incline Press	1 x 8, 2 x 6
DB Lying Flys	3 x 10
DB Front Raises	3 x 10
DB Lateral Raises	3 x 10
DB Bent-over Lateral Raises	3 x 10 SS
Bench Dips	3 x 15

DB Curls	3 x 8	DB Hammer Curls	3 x 8
Rice Routine		Rice Routine	
Abdominal #1		Med Ball Abdominal	
Plyometrics #'s	2, 7, 8, 18	Plyometrics #'s	19, 25, 29, 32

Day 2		Day 4	
Rotator Cuff Warm-up	x 2	Rotator Cuff Warm-up	x 2
Pull-ups	3 x 10	Incline Pull-ups	3 x 12
Twisting Back Extension	3 x 20 TS	Good Mornings	3 x 15 SS
Torso Twists	3 x 20	Hang Snatch	3 x 5
Power Snatch	1 x 8, 3 x 6	DB Lunges	3 x 8
Power Squat	1 x 8, 3 x 6	Leg Extensions	3 x 10
Seated Calves	3 x 25	Leg Curls	3 x 10 SS
Lat Pull-downs	3 x 10	Standing Calves, Single	3 x 20
Pull-overs	3 x 10	Straight Lat Pull-downs	3 x 10
Hip Routine		Hip Routine	
Back Stabilization		Back Stabilization	
Med Ball Routine #'s	9, 12. 14, 16	Med Ball Routine #'s	11, 13, 16

Peak/Transition Phase

Day 1		Day 3	
Rotator Cuff Warm-up	x 2	Rotator Cuff Warm-up	x 2
Decline Push-ups	1 x 20	Push-ups	1 x 20
Reverse Back Extension	1 x 20	Back Extension	1 x 20
DB Bench Press	1 x 8, 1 x 6, 2 x 4	DB Incline Press	1 x 8, 1 x 6, 1 x 4
DB Incline Flys	3 x 10	DB Lying Flys	3 x 8
DB Military Press	3 x 6	DB Front Raises	2 x 10
Med Ball Over-head Pass	3 x 10 SS	DB Lateral Raises	2 x 10 TS
Rear Deltoid Pulls	2 x 10	DB Bent-over Lateral Raises	2 x 10
Dips	2 x 15	Bench Dips	2 x 20
DB Curls	3 x 8	DB Hammer Curls	3 x 8
Abdominal #1		Med Ball Abdominal	
Plyometrics #'s	1, 7, 18	Plyometrics #'s	26, 30, 32

Day 2		Day 4	
Rotator Cuff Warm-up	x 2	Rotator Cuff Warm-up	x 2
Pull-ups	1 x 12	Incline Pull-ups	1 x 15
Twisting Back Extension	1 x 20	Good Mornings	1 x 15
Torso Twists	1 x 20	High Pulls	2 x 8
Power Snatch	1 x 8, 1 x 6, 2 x 4	Box Jumps	2 x 10 SS

Power Squat	1 x 8, 1 x 6, 2 x 4	Leg Extensions, Single	2 x 10
Single Leg Box Jumps	4 x 10 SS	Leg Curls, Single	2 x 10
Seated Calves	2 x 25	Standing Calves, Single	2 x 20
Lat Pull-downs	2 x 10	Straight Lat Pull-downs	3 x 10
Pull-overs	2 x 10	Hip Routine	
Hip Routine		Back Stabilization	
Back Stabilization			

TRACK AND FIELD (POLE VAULTERS) (IN-SEASON PHASE)

Day 1		Day 2	
Rotator Cuff Warm-up	x 2	Rotator Cuff Warm-up	x 2
Decline Push-ups	1 x 20	Pull-ups	1 x 12
Reverse Back Extension	1 x 20	Twisting Back Extension	1 x 20
DB Bench Press	3 x 8	Torso Twists	1 x 20
DB Incline Flys	2 x 15	*Power Snatch Combo	3 x 5
DB Military Press	3 x 8	Leg Extensions	2 x 12
Med Ball Over-head Pass	3 x 10 SS	Leg Curls	2 x 12 SS
Rear Deltoid Pulls	2 x 10	Straight Lat Pull-downs	2 x 12
Dips	2 x 15	Hip Routine	
DB Curls	3 x 8	Back Stabilization	
Abdominal #1			

*Power snatch combo: Perform power snatch, overhead squat (keep bar in overhead position while performing a squat), and push press for repetition.

TRACK AND FIELD (SPRINTERS)

Introductory Phase

Day 1		Day 3	
Rotator Cuff Warm-up	x 1	Rotator Cuff Warm-up	x 1
Push-ups	2 x 10	Dips	2 x 10
DB Lying Flys	2 x 15 SS	DB Incline Flys	2 x 15 SS
Bench Press	3 x 15	Incline Press	3 x 15
DB Upright Rows	3 x 15	Cable Front Raises	3 x 15
DB Reverse Lateral Raises	3 x 15 SS	Cable Lateral Raises	3 x 15
Rear Deltoid Pulls	3 x 15	DB Bent-over Front Raises	3 x 15
DB Incline Curls	3 x 10	E-Z Bar Curls	3 x 15
Straight Bar Curls	3 x 15	DB Hammer Curls	3 x 12
DB Lying Tricep Extension	3 x 15 SS	Tricep Push-down	3 x 15 SS

DB Tricep Kickback	3 x 12	DB Tricep Extension	3 x 12
Abdominal #1		Abdominal #2	

Day 2		**Day 4**	
Rotator Cuff Warm-up	x 1	Rotator Cuff Warm-up	x 1
Pull-ups	3 x 5	Incline Pull-ups	3 x 8
DB Stiff Leg Dead Lift	3 x 10	Good Mornings	3 x 10 SS
High Pulls	3 x 10	Hang Cleans	3 x 8
Hang Cleans	2 x 10	Power Squat	3 x 15
DB Step-ups	3 x 10	Leg Extensions	3 x 15
Leg Curls	3 x 10 SS	Leg Curls	3 x 15 SS
Seated Calves	3 x 25	Standing Calves	3 x 25
DB Pull-overs	3 x 15	Seated Rows	3 x 15
T-Bar Rows	3 x 15	Lat Pull-downs	3 x 15
Hip Routine		Hip Routine	
Back Stabilization		Back Stabilization	

Strength Phase

Day 1		**Day 3**	
Rotator Cuff Warm-up	x 1	Rotator Cuff Warm-up	x 1
Push-ups	2 x 12	Dips	2 x 12
Bench Press	3 x 10	Incline Press	3 x 10
DB Lying Flys	3 x 10	DB Incline Flys	3 x 10
DB Standing Military	3 x 10	DB Front Raises	3 x 10
DB Upright Rows	3 x 10	DB Lateral Raises	3 x 10
DB Reverse Lateral Raises	3 x 10 SS	DB Bent-over Lateral Raises	3 x 10
DB Hammer Curls	3 x 10	E-Z Bar Curls	3 x 12
Straight Bar Curls	3 x 10	Straight Bar Curls	3 x 12
DB Tricep Kickback	3 x 10 SS	Bench Dips	3 x 10
Tricep Push-down	3 x 10	DB Lying Tricep Extension	3 x 10
Abdominal #1		Med Ball Abdominal	

Day 2		**Day 4**	
Rotator Cuff Warm-ups	x 1	Rotator Cuff Warm-ups	x 1
Pull-ups	2 x 8	Incline Pull-ups	2 x 10
High Pulls	2 x 8	Good Mornings	2 x 10 SS
Hang Cleans	3 x 8	DB Hang Cleans	3 x 8
Leg Extensions	3 x 10	Front Squat	3 x 10
Leg Curls	3 x 10 SS	Leg Extensions	3 x 10
Seated Calves	3 x 25	Leg Curls	3 x 10 SS
Seated Rows	3 x 10	Standing Calves	3 x 25
Lat Pull-downs	3 x 10	DB One Arm Rows	3 x 10

Hip Routine
Back Stabilization

DB Pull-overs   3 x 10
Hip Routine
Back Stabilization

Power Phase

Day 1	
Rotator Cuff Warm-up	x 1
Push-ups	2 x 15
Bench Press	1 x 8, 2 x 6
DB Lying Flys	3 x 10
DB Military	3 x 8
Upright Row	3 x 8
Rear Deltoid Pulls	3 x 10
DB Incline Curls	3 x 8
Cable Curls	3 x 10
DB Tricep Extension	3 x 8 SS
Tricep Push-down	3 x 10
Abdominal #1	
Plyometrics #'s	2, 18, 19, 20

Day 3	
Rotator Cuff Warm-ups	x 1
Dips	2 x 15
Incline Press	1 x 8, 2 x 6
DB Incline Flys	3 x 10
DB Front Raises	3 x 8
DB Lateral Raises	3 x 8
DB Bent-over Lat Raises	3 x 8
DB Hammer Curls	3 x 10
Straight Bar Curls	3 x 10
DB Tricep Kickback	3 x 10
Bench Dips	3 x 15
Med Ball Abdominal	
Plyometrics #'s	25, 27, 28, 30, 32

Day 2	
Rotator Cuff Warm-ups	x 1
Pull-ups	2 x 10
DB Stiff Leg Dead Lift	2 x 10 SS
Power Cleans	1 x 8, 2 x 6
DB Step-ups	3 x 8
DB Squat	3 x 8
Seated Calves	3 x 25
Seated Rows	3 x 10
Lat Pull-downs	3 x 10
Hip Routine	
Back Stabilization	
Ladder	1 set

Day 4	
Rotator Cuff Warm-ups	x 1
Pull-ups	2 x 10
Good Mornings	2 x 10 SS
DB Hang Cleans	2 x 8
Power Squat	1 x 8, 2 x 6
DB Jump Squat	3 x 10
Leg Curls	3 x 10 SS
Standing Calves	3 x 25
DB One Arm Rows	3 x 10
DB Pull-overs	3 x 10
Hip Routine	
Back Stabilization	

Peak/Transition Phase

Day 1	
Rotator Cuff Warm-up	x 1
Push-ups	2 x 15
DB Lying Flys	2 x 10
Bench Press	1 x 8, 1 x 6, 2 x 4
Upright Rows	3 x 8

Day 3	
Rotator Cuff Warm-up	x 1
Dips	2 x 15
DB Incline Flys	3 x 10
Incline Press	1 x 8, 1 x 6, 2 x 4
DB Reverse Lateral Raises	3 x 10

Rear Deltoid Pulls	3 x 8	DB Bent-over Front Raises	3 x 10
DB Incline Curls	3 x 8	DB Hammer Curls	3 x 10
Tricep Push-down	3 x 10	DB Tricep Kickback	3 x 10
Abdominal #1		Med Ball Abdominal	
Plyometrics #'s	1, 3, 9, 19	Plyometrics #'s	20,26, 29, 32

Day 2		Day 4	
Rotator Cuff Warm-ups	x 1	Rotator Cuff Warm-ups	x 1
Pull-ups	2 x 10	Pull-ups	2 x 10
DB Stiff Leg Dead Lift	2 x 10 SS	Good Mornings	2 x 10 SS
Power Cleans	1 x 8, 1 x 6, 2 x 4	DB Hang Cleans	2 x 8
Box Jumps	4 x 10 SS	Quarter Squat	1 x 8, 1 x 6, 2 x 4
DB Walking Lunges	2 x 10	Squat Jumps	4 x 10 SS
Single Leg 6-Iinch Box Jumps	2 x 10 SS	Leg Curl	3 x 10
Seated Calves	2 x 25	Standing Calves, Single	3 x 25
Seated Rows	3 x 10	DB One Arm Rows	3 x 8
Hip Routine		Hip Routine	
Back Stabilization		Back Stabilization	
Ladder	1 set	Ladder	1 set

TRACK AND FIELD (SPRINTERS) (IN-SEASON PHASE)

Day 1		Day 2	
Rotator Cuff Warm-up	x 1	Rotator Cuff Warm-up	x 1
Push-ups	2 x 15	Pull-ups	2 x 10
Good Mornings	2 x 20 SS	Torso Twists	2 x 20 SS
DB Bench Press	2 x 10	DB Hang Cleans	2 x 8
DB Incline Flys	2 x 10 SS	Squat Jumps	2 x 10 SS
DB Upright Rows	3 x 8	Quarter Squat	3 x 8
Leg Extensions	2 x 15	Single Leg 6-Inch Box Jumps	3 x 10 SS
Leg Curls	2 x 15 TS	Lat Pull-downs	3 x 12
Seated Calves	2 x 25	DB Reverse Lateral Raises	3 x 12 SS
DB Tricep Kickback	3 x 10	DB Hammer Curls	3 x 10
Hip Routine		Hip Routine	
Abdominal #1		Abdominal #2	
Back Stabilization		Back Stabilization	

TRACK AND FIELD (THROWERS)

Introductory Phase

Day 1	
Rotator Cuff Warm-up	x 2
Push-ups	3 x 10
DB Lying Flys	3 x 10 SS
Bench Press	4 x 10
Incline Press	3 x 10
Military Press	3 x 10
Upright Rows	3 x 15
DB Lying Tricep Extension	3 x 15
Bench Dips	3 x 10
Abdominal #1	
Reverse Back Extension	3 x 10

Day 3	
Rotator Cuff Warm-up	x 2
Decline Push-ups	3 x 10
DB Incline Flys	3 x 15 SS
DB Bench Press	3 x 10
DB Incline Press	3 x 10
DB Front Raises	3 x 15
DB Lateral Raises	3 x 15
Tricep Push-down	3 x 15
DB Tricep Extension	3 x 15
Abdominal #2	
Reverse Back Extension	3 x 10

Day 2	
Rotator Cuff Warm-up	x 1
Pull-ups	3 x 5
Good Mornings	3 x 15 SS
High Pulls	3 x 10
Hang Cleans	3 x 8
Dead Lift	3 x 8
DB Pull-overs	3 x 15
Bent-over Barbell Rows	3 x 15
DB Curls	3 x 10
Straight Bar Curls	3 x 15
Hip Routine	
Back Stabilization	

Day 4	
Rotator Cuff Warm-up	x 1
DB Stiff Leg Dead Lift	3 x 15
Leg Curls	3 x 15 SS
Power Squat	3 x 10
Lunges	3 x 10
Power Shrugs	3 x 10
Seated Rows	3 x 15
Straight Lat Pull-downs	3 x 15
DB Hammer Curls	3 x 10
Cable Curls	3 x 15
Hip Routine	
Back Stabilization	

Strength Phase

Day 1	
Rotator Cuff Warm-up	x 2
Push-ups	3 x 12
DB Lying Flys	3 x 10 SS
Bench Press	1 x 10, 3 x 8
Incline Press	1 x 10, 2 x 8
Military Press	3 x 8

Day 3	
Rotator Cuff Warm-up	x 2
Decline Push-ups	3 x 12
DB Incline Flys	3 x 12 SS
DB Bench Press	3 x 8
DB Incline Press	3 x 8
Upright Rows	3 x 10

DB Reverse Lateral Raises	3 x 10
Rear Deltoid Pulls	3 x 10
DB Tricep Extension	3 x 10
Bench Dips	3 x 12
Abdominal #1	

DB Bent-over Lateral Raises	3 x 10
Tricep Push-down	3 x 10
DB Lying Tricep Extension	3 x 10
Med Ball Abdominal	
Slide Board	3 x 30

Day 2

Rotator Cuff Warm-up	x 1
Pull-ups	3 x 8
Good Mornings	3 x 10 SS
High Pulls	2 x 8
Power Cleans	1 x 8, 3 x 6
Dead Lift	3 x 8
DB Pull-overs	3 x 10
Seated Rows	3 x 10
DB Incline Curls	3 x 10
Cable Curls	3 x 12
Hip Routine	
Back Stabilization	

Day 4

Rotator Cuff Warm-up	x 1
Back Extension	3 x 15
Incline Pull-ups	3 x 10 SS
Squat	1 x 8, 3 x 6
Push Press	3 x 8
Power Shrugs	3 x 8
DB One Arm Rows	3 x 10
Lat Pull-downs	3 x 15
DB Hammer Curls	3 x 10
Straight Bar Curls	3 x 10
Hip Routine	
Back Stabilization	

Power Phase

Day 1

Rotator Cuff Warm-up	x 2
Push-ups	3 x 15
DB Lying Flys	3 x 10 SS
Bench Press	1 x 8, 1 x 6, 2 x 4
Incline Press	1 x 8, 1 x 6, 1 x 4
Military Press	4 x 6
Upright Rows	3 x 8
DB Lying Tricep Extension	3 x 10
DB Tricep Extension	3 x 10
Abdominal #1	
Reverse Back Extension	3 x 10
Plyometrics #'s	2, 7, 8, 11

Day 3

Rotator Cuff Warm-up	x 2
Decline Push-ups	3 x 15
DB Incline Flys	3 x 10 SS
DB Bench Press	4 x 6
Close Grip Bench Press	3 x 8
DB Bent-over Front Raises	3 x 10
DB Bent-over Lateral Raises	3 x 10
Tricep Push-down	3 x 10
Reverse Tricep Extension	3 x 10
Med Ball Abdominal	
Reverse Back Extension	3 x 10
Plyometrics #'s	18, 19, 28, 32

Day 2

Rotator Cuff Warm-up	x 1
Pull-ups	3 x 10
Good Mornings	3 x 10 SS
Power Cleans	1 x 8, 1 x 6, 2 x 4
Push Press	4 x 6

Day 4

Rotator Cuff Warm-up	x 1
Incline Pull-ups	3 x 15
Torso Twists	3 x 20 SS
Power Squat	1 x 8, 1 x 6, 2 x 4
Dead Lift	3 x 6

Power Shrugs	3 x 6	Reverse Lunges	3 x 8
DB Pull-overs	3 x 8	DB One Arm Rows	3 x 10
Seated Rows	3 x 8	Lat Pull-downs	3 x 10
DB Incline Curls	3 x 10	Straight Bar Curls	3 x 10
Hip Routine		Hip Routine	
Back Stabilization		Back Stabilization	
Med Ball Routine #'s	2, 5, 6, 10	Med Ball Routine #'s	11, 14, 15, 16

Peak/Transition Phase

Day 1

Rotator Cuff Warm-up	x 2
Push-ups	2 x 15
DB Lying Flys	2 x 10 SS
Bench Press	1 x 8, 1 x 6, 1 x 4, 2 x 2
Incline Press	1 x 8, 1 x 5, 1 x 3
Military Press	3 x 5
Med Ball Supine Drops	3 x 10 SS
Upright Rows	2 x 8
DB Lying Tricep Extension	3 x 8
DB Tricep Extension	3 x 8
Abdominal #1	
Plyometrics #'s	1, 7, 10, 13

Day 3

Rotator Cuff Warm-up	x 2
Decline Push-ups	2 x 15
DB Incline Flys	3 x 10 SS
DB Bench Press	3 x 5
Close Grip Bench Press	2 x 8
DB Bent-over Front Raises	3 x 10
Med Ball Over-head Pass	3 x 10
DB Tricep Extension	2 x 10
Tricep Push-down	3 x 10
Abdominal #2	
Plyometrics #'s	20, 27, 29, 32

Day 2

Rotator Cuff Warm-up	
Pull-ups	2 x 10
Good Mornings	2 x 10 SS
Power Cleans	1 x 8, 1 x 6, 1 x 4, 2 x 2
Push Press	3 x 5
Med Ball Chest Pass	3 x 10 SS
Seated Rows	2 x 8
DB Pull-overs	3 x 8
DB Hammer Curls	3 x 10
Hip Routine	
Back Stabilization	
Med Ball Routine #'s	6, 7, 9

Day 4

Rotator Cuff Warm-up	x 1
Back Extension	3 x 20
Torso Twists	3 x 20 SS
Power Squat	1 x 8, 1 x 5, 2 x 3
Dead Lift	2 x 5
Reverse Lunges	2 x 8
Single Leg 6-Iinch Box Jumps	2 x 10 SS
DB One Arm Rows	2 x 10
Lat Pull-downs	3 x 10
Straight Bar Curls	3 x 10
Hip Routine	
Back Stabilization	
Med Ball Routine #'s	11, 14, 15, 16

TRACK AND FIELD (THROWERS) (IN-SEASON PHASE)

Day 1		Day 2	
Rotator Cuff Warm-up	x 1	Rotator Cuff Warm-ups	x 1
Push-ups	2 x 15	Incline Pull-ups	2 x 10
Reverse Back Extension	2 x 10 TS	Twisting Back Extension	2 x 20 TS
Torso Twists	2 x 20	Torso Twists	2 x 20
Bench Press	3 x 8	*Power Clean Combo	2 x 5
Med Ball Chest Pass	3 x 10 SS	Single Leg 6-Inch Box Jumps	2 x 10 SS
DB Incline Press	3 x 8	Barbell Bent-over Row	3 x 10
Upright Rows	2 x 10	Pull-over	3 x 10
Rear Deltoid Pulls	3 x 10	DB Hammer Curl	3 x 10
DB Lying Tricep Extension	3 x 10	Back Stabilization	
Abdominal #1			

* Power clean combo: Perform power clean, front squat, push press for one combo repetition.

VOLLEYBALL

Introductory Phase

Day 1		Day 3	
Rotator Cuff Warm-ups	x 2	Rotator Cuff Warm-ups	x 2
Decline Push-ups	3 x 10	Push-ups	3 x 10
Torso Twists	3 x 20	DB Side Bends	3 x 10
DB Bench Press	3 x 15	DB Incline Press	3 x 15
DB Lying Flys	3 x 15	DB Incline Flys	3 x 15
DB Standing Military	3 x 12	Cable Upright Rows	3 x 15
DB Reverse Lateral Raises	3 x 15	DB Lateral Raises	3 x 15
Rear Deltoid Pulls	3 x 15	DB Bent-over Lat Raises	3 x 15
Bench Dips	2 x 10	Dips	2 x 5
DB Hammer Curls	2 x 10	DB Incline Curls	2 x 10
Abdominal #1		Abdominal #2	

Day 2		Day 4	
Rotator Cuff Warm-up	x 1	Rotator Cuff Warm-up	x 1
Pull-ups	3 x 5	Incline Pull-ups	3 x 8
Twisting Back Extension	3 x 20	Back Extension	3 x 20

High Pulls	3 x 10	DB Hang Cleans	3 x 12
Leg Sled	3 x 15	Power Squat	3 x 12
Lateral Lunges	3 x 10	Walking Lunges	2 x 20
Leg Curls	3 x 15	Leg Extensions, Single	2 x 15 TS
Straight Lat Pull-downs	3 x 15	Leg Curls, Single	2 x 15
Seated Rows	3 x 15	DB Pull-overs	3 x 15
Seated Calves	2 x 25	Standing Calves	2 x 50
Hip Routine		Hip Routine	
Back Stabilization		Back Stabilization	

Strength Phase

Day 1

Rotator Cuff Warm-up	x 2		
Decline Push-ups	3 x 12		
Torso Twists	3 x 20		
DB Bench Press	3 x 10		
DB Lying Flys	3 x 10		
DB Push Press	3 x 10		
DB Front Raise	3 x 12		
Rear Deltoid PullS	3 x 12		
Bench Dips	2 x 12		
DB Hammer Curl	2 x 10		
Abdominal #1			
Slide Board	3 x 30		

Day 3

Rotator Cuff Warm-up	x 2
Push-ups	3 x 15
DB Side Bends	3 x 10
DB Incline Press	3 x 10
DB Incline Flys	3 x 10
Cable Upright Row	3 x 12
DB Bent-over Front Raise	3 x 12
DB Bent-over Lateral Raise	3 x 15
Dips	2 x 8
DB Incline Curls	2 x 10
Med Ball Abdominal	
Slide Board	3 x 30

Day 2

Rotator Cuff Warm-up	
Pull-ups	3 x 8
Twisting Back Extension	3 x 20
High Pulls	3 x 8
Leg Sled	3 x 10
4-way Lunges	2 x 10
Leg Curls	3 x 10
Straight Lat Pull-downs	3 x 12
Seated Rows	3 x 12
Seated Calves	2 x 30
Hip Routine	
Back Stabilization	

Day 4

Rotator Cuff Warm-ups	
Incline Pull-ups	3 x 10
Reverse Back Extension	3 x 20
DB Hang Cleans	3 x 10
Squat	3 x 10
Leg Extensions	3 x 10
Leg Curls	3 x 10
Barbell Bent-over Rows	3 x 12
DB Pull-overs	3 x 12
Standing Calves	2 x 50
Hip Routine	
Back Stabilization	

Power Phase

Day 1			Day 3		
Rotator Cuff Warm-up	x 2		Rotator Cuff Warm-up	x 2	
Decline Push-ups	3 x 15		Med Ball Push-ups	3 x 10	
Torso Twists	3 x 20 SS		DB Side Bends	3 x 10	
DB Bench Press	3 x 8		DB Incline Press	3 x 8	
DB Lying Flys	3 x 10		DB Incline Flys	3 x 10	
DB Push Press	3 x 8		Cable Upright Rows	3 x 10	
DB Front Raises	3 x 10		DB Bent-over Front Raises	3 x 10	
Rear Deltoid Pulls	3 x 10		DB Bent-over Lat Raises	3 x 10	
Bench Dips	2 x 15		Dips	2 x 10	
DB Hammer Curls	2 x 10		Straight Bar Curls	2 x 10	
Med Ball Abdominal			Abdominal #2		
Slide Board	3 x 60		Slide Board	3 x 30	
Plyometrics #'s	2, 4, 6, 7		Plyometrics #'s	9, 11, 12, 14	

Day 2			Day 4		
Rotator Cuff Warm-up	x 1		Rotator Cuff Warm-up		
Pull-ups	3 x 10		Pull-ups	3 x 10	
Twisting Back Extension	3 x 20		Reverse Back Extension	3 x 20	
Power Cleans	3 x 8		Hang Cleans	3 x 8	
Leg Sled	1 x 8, 3 x 6		Quarter Squat	3 x 8	
DB Squat	2 x 10		Leg Extensions, Single	2 x 10	
Leg Curls	2 x 10		Leg Curls, Single	2 x 10	
Straight Lat Pull-downs	3 x 10		DB One Arm Rows	3 x 10	
Seated Rows	3 x 10		DB Pull-overs	3 x 10	
Seated Calves	2 x 40		Standing Calves, Single	2 x 50	
Back Stabilization			Back Stabilization		
Hip Routine			Hip Routine		
Med Ball Routine #'s	5, 9, 12		Med Ball Routine #'s	13, 14, 16	

Peak/Transition Phase

Day 1			Day 3		
Rotator Cuff Warm-up	x 2		Rotator Cuff Warm-ups	x 2	
Decline Push-ups	2 x 15		Med Ball Push-ups	2 x 10	
Torso Twists	2 x 20		DB Side Bends	2 x 10	
DB Bench Press	1 x 8, 3 x 6		DB Incline Press	3 x 8	
Med Ball Chest Pass	4 x 10 SS		Med Ball Over-head Pass	3 x 10 SS	
DB Lying Flys	3 x 10		DB Incline Flys	3 x 10	

DB Push Press	3 x 8	Cable Upright Rows	3 x 10
DB Front Raises	3 x 10	DB Bent-over Front Raises	3 x 10
Rear Deltoid Pulls	3 x 10	DB Bent-over Lateral Raises	3 x 10
Bench Dips	2 x 20	Dips	2 x 10
DB Hammer Curls	2 x 10	Straight Bar Curls	2 x 10
Med Ball Abdominal		Abdominal #2	
Slide Board	1 x 60	Slide Board	3 x 20
Plyometrics #'s	3, 9, 12, 16	Plyometrics #'s	10, 14, 17, 20

Day 2		Day 4	
Rotator Cuff Warm-ups	x 1	Rotator Cuff Warm-ups	x 1
Pull-ups	2 x 10	Pull-ups	2 x 10
Twisting Back Extension	2 x 20	Back Extension	2 x 20
Power Cleans	3 x 8	Hang Cleans	3 x 8
Lateral Cone Hops	3 x 10 SS	Depth Jumps	3 x 5 SS
Leg Sled	1 x 8, 3 x 6	Quarter Squat	3 x 8
DB Squat	2 x 10	Leg Extension, Single	2 x 10
Squat Jumps	2 x 10 SS	Leg Curls, Single	2 x 10 SS
Straight Lat Pull-downs	3 x 10	DB One Arm Rows	3 x 10
Seated Rows	3 x 10	DB Pull-overs	3 x 10
Back Stabilization		Hip Routine	
Med Ball Routine #'s	5, 7, 9	Med Ball Routine #'s	12, 14, 16

VOLLEYBALL (IN-SEASON PHASE)

Day 1		Day 2	
Rotator Cuff Warm-up	x 2	Rotator Cuff Warm-up	x 2
Twisting Back Extension	2 x 20	Prone Back Extension	2 x 20
Torso Twists	2 x 20 TS	DB Side Bends	2 x 10 TS
Med Ball Push-ups	2 x 15	Incline Pull-ups	2 x 10
*DB Hang Clean Combo	2 x 5	Quarter Squat	3 x 8
Depth Jumps	2 x 5 SS	Lateral Cone Hops	3 x 10 SS
Leg Extensions, Single	2 x 10	Leg Curls, Single	2 x 10
DB Lying Flys	2 x 15	DB Incline Flys	2 x 15
Med-Ball Over-head Pass	2 x 10 SS	Cable Upright Rows	2 x 10 SS
DB Bent-over Front Raises	2 x 10	DB Bent-over Lateral Raises	2 x 10
Bench Dips	2 x 15	DB Hammer Curls	2 x 10
Back Stabilization		Back Stabilization	
Abdominal #1		Abdominal #2	

* DB Hang clean combo: Perform DB hang clean, DB push press, and DB squat for one repetition.

WRESTLING

Introductory Phase

Day 1	
Rotator Cuff Warm-up	x 2
Neck (4-Way)	1 x 10
Decline Push-ups	3 x 10
DB Incline Flys	3 x 15 SS
DB Bench Press	3 x 15
Upright Rows	3 x 15
DB Reverse Lateral Raises	3 x 15 SS
Rear Deltoid Pulls	3 x 15
Straight Bar Curls	3 x 15
DB Hammer Curls	3 x 10
Rice Routine	
Abdominal #1	

Day 2	
Rotator Cuff Warm-up	x 1
Pull-ups	3 x 5
Back Extension	3 x 10
Torso Twists	3 x 20 SS
High Pulls	3 x 10
Push Press	3 x 8
DB Step-ups	3 x 10
Leg Curls	3 x 10 SS
Seated Calves	3 x 25
DB One Arm Rows	3 x 15
Barbell Bent-over Rows	3 x 15
Hip Routine	
Back Stabilization	

Day 3	
Rotator Cuff Warm-up	x 2
Neck (4-Way)	1 x 10
Push-ups	3 x 12
Cable Flys	3 x 15 SS
DB Incline Press	3 x 15
DB Front Raises	3 x 15
DB Lateral Raises	3 x 15
DB Bent-over Lateral Raises	3 x 15
Dips	3 x 10
DB Lying Tricep Extension	3 x 15
Rice Routine	
Abdominal #2	

Day 4	
Rotator Cuff Warm-up	x 1
Incline Pull-ups	3 x 10
Reverse Back Extension	3 x 10
Torso Twists	3 x 20 SS
Hang Cleans	3 x 10
Power Squat	3 x 15
Leg Extensions	2 x 20
Leg Curls	2 x 20
Standing Calves	2 x 20
Straight Lat Pull-downs	3 x 15
Seated Rows	3 x 15
Hip Routine	
Back Stabilization	

Strength Phase

Day 1	
Rotator Cuff Warm-ups	x 2
Neck (4-Way)	1 x 10
DB Bench Press	3 x 10

Day 3	
Rotator Cuff Warm-ups	x 2
Neck (4-Way)	1 x 10
DB Incline Press	3 x 10

Decline Push-ups	3 x 12	Push-ups	3 x 15
DB Incline Flys	3 x 12 SS	Cable Flys	3 x 12 SS
DB Upright Rows	3 x 12	DB Standing Military Press	3 x 10
DB Reverse Lateral Raises	3 x 12	DB Lateral Raise	3 x 12
Rear Deltoid Pulls	3 x 12	DB Bent-over Front Raise	3 x 12
DB Curls	3 x 12	Dips	3 x 12
Straight Bar Curls	3 x 10	DB Lying Tricep Extension	3 x 10
Rice Routine		Rice Routine	
Abdominal #1		Med Ball Abdominal	

Day 2		Day 4	
Rotator Cuff Warm-up	x 1	Rotator Cuff Warm-up	x 1
Pull-ups	3 x 8	Incline Pull-ups	3 x 15
Reverse Back Extension	3 x 15	Twisting Back Extension	3 x 10
Torso Twists	3 x 20 SS	Torso Twists	3 x 20 SS
High Pulls	3 x 8	Power Cleans	3 x 8
Push Press	3 x 8	Front Squat	3 x 10
Walking Lunges	3 x 10	Leg Extensions, Single	2 x 15
Leg Curls	3 x 10 SS	Leg Curls, Single	2 x 15
Seated Calves	3 x 30	Standing Calves, Single	2 x 25
Lat Pull-downs	3 x 12	Straight Lat Pull-downs	3 x 12
Barbell Bent-over Rows	3 x 12	Pull-overs	3 x 12
Hip Routine		Hip Routine	
Back Stabilization		Back Stabilization	

Power Phase

Day 1		Day 3	
Rotator Cuff Warm-up	x 2	Rotator Cuff Warm-up	x 2
Prone Neck Extension	2 x 30	Supine Neck Flexion	2 x 30
*Swiss Ball DB Bench Press	3 x 8	DB Incline Press	4 x 8
Decline Push-ups	3 x 15	Med Ball Push-ups	3 x 10
DB Incline Flys	3 x 10	*Swiss Ball DB Flys	3 x 10
Upright Rows	3 x 10	DB Standing Military Press	3 x 8
DB Front Raises	3 x 10	DB Lateral Raises	3 x 10
Rear Deltoid Pulls	3 x 10	DB Bent-over Front Raises	3 x 10
DB Hammer Curls	3 x 10	Dips	3 x 15
Straight Bar Curls	3 x 10	Tricep Push-downs	3 x 10
Abdominal #1		Med Ball Abdominal	
Plyometrics #'s	1, 11, 12, 16, 20	Plyometrics #'s	22, 23, 30, 32

* Swiss ball lift: Perform lift in bridge position on ball. Shoulder blades are on ball, feet on floor.

Day 2	
Rotator Cuff Warm-up	x 1
Pull-ups	3 x 10
Reverse Back Extension	3 x 20
High Pulls	3 x 8
Quarter Squat	3 x 8
Squat Jumps	3 x 10 SS
Seated Calves	2 x 30
DB One Arm Rows	3 x 10
T-Bar Rows	3 x 10
Back Stabilization	
Med Ball Routine #'s	4, 6, 12, 14

Day 4	
Rotator Cuff Warm-up	x 1
Incline Pull-ups	3 x 20
Twisting Back Extension	3 x 10
*Power Clean Combo	3 x 5
Leg Curls	3 x 10
Single Leg 6-Inch Box Jumps	3 x 10 SS
Standing Calves	2 x 25
Seated Rows	3 x 10
Pull-overs	3 x 10
Back Stabilization	
Med Ball Routine #'s	9, 13, 15, 16

*Power clean combo: Perform one repetition power clean, one repetition front squat, one repetition push press for one combo repetition.

Peak/Transition Phase

Day 1	
Rotator Cuff Warm-ups	x 1
Prone Neck Extension	2 x 30
*Swiss Ball DB Bench Press	4 x 6
Med Ball Chest Pass	4 x 5 SS
Decline Push-ups	2 x 20
DB Incline Flys	2 x 8
Upright Rows	2 x 10
Rear Deltoid Pull	2 x 10
DB Hammer Curls	3 x 10
Abdominal #2	
Plyometrics #'s	9, 12, 22, 23

Day 3	
Rotator Cuff Warm-ups	x 1
Supine Neck Flexion	2 x 30
DB Incline Press	3 x 5
Med Ball Over-head Pass	3 x 5 SS
Med Ball Push-ups	2 x 12
*Swiss Ball DB Flys	2 x 10 SS
DB Standing Military Press	3 x 6
DB Bent-over Front Raises	2 x 10
Dips	3 x 15
Med Ball Abdominal	
Plyometrics #'s	26, 27, 29, 31, 32

* Swiss ball lifts: Perform lift in bridge position. Shoulder blades on ball, feet on floor.

Day 2	
Rotator Cuff Warm-up	x 1
Pull-ups	2 x 12
Reverse Back Extension	2 x 20
Med Ball Wood Choppers	2 x 10 SS
High Pulls	2 x 8
Quarter Squat	3 x 8
Squat Jumps	3 x 8 SS
Seated Calves	2 x 30
T-Bar Rows	2 x 10
Back Stabilization	

Day 4	
Rotator Cuff Warm-up	x 1
Incline Pull-ups	2 x 20
Twisting Back Extension	2 x 10
Med Ball Twists	2 x 10 SS
*Power Clean Combo	2 x 5
Leg Curls	2 x 10
Single Leg 6-Inch Box Jumps	2 x 10 SS
Standing Calves	2 x 25
Pull-overs	2 x 10
Back Stabilization	

*Power clean combo: Perform power clean, front squat, and push press for one combo repetition.

WRESTLING (IN SEASON PHASE)

Day 1		Day 2	
Rotator Cuff Warm-up		Rotator Cuff Warm-ups	x 1
Med Ball Push-ups	2 x 15	Pull-ups	2 x 10
Prone Neck Extension	2 x 30 TS	Supine Neck Flexion	2 x 30 TS
Med Ball Wood Choppers	2 x 20	Med Ball Twists	2 x 20
Hang Cleans	3 x 8	Hang Snatch	3 x 5
Leg Curls	3 x 8 SS	Squat Jumps	3 x 10 SS
*Swiss Ball DB Bench Press	3 x 8	DB Incline Press	3 x 8
Med Ball Chest Pass	3 x 5 SS	Swiss Ball DB Military Press	2 x 8
DB Bent-over Front Raises	2 x 12	Rear Deltoid Pulls	3 x 10
DB Reverse Lateral Raises	2 x 12 SS	DB Hammer Curls	3 x 10
Dips	2 x 10	Med Ball Abdominal	
Back Stabilization			

*Swiss ball lifts: Perform lift in bridge position. Shoulder blades on ball, feet on floor.

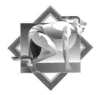

Appendix

Weightlifting Descriptions

Abdominal: See program.

Alternating scissor jumps: See plyometric program.

Ankle hops: See plyometric program.

Back extension (body weight): Prone on the floor (pad/pillow under hips) or apparatus, hands behind the back for beginners, working toward the head for advanced, torso stable and feet secure. Extend back until the chest is no longer touching the floor or parallel with the floor if on an apparatus, control descent (Figure A-1).

Back stabilization: See descriptions and figures.

Bench dips (body weight): Hands on bench, elbows extended, shoulders slightly hyperextended (behind torso) and internally rotated, knees slightly flexed for beginners working toward full extension. For advanced, torso stable, exhale and slowly flex elbows to 90 degrees, inhale and extend elbows fully. Do not allow hips to sag during exercise.

Bench press (dumbbell [DB]/barbell): Straddle bench, feet on the ground, knees flexed to 90 degrees; head, shoulders, and hips on bench at all times, overhand grip wider than shoulder width. Keep wrists tight and in line with the elbows. Inhale and, with control, lower the barbell/DB to breast line, exhale while pushing upward and back to eye level. Barbell/DB should execute a slightly curved descent and ascent. At completion of ascent, the wrists should still be in line with the extended elbows.

Bent-over front raise (DB): Feet shoulder width apart, knees slightly flexed, hips flexed to 90 degrees, chest and chin up, and keep torso stable (contract abdominals, gluteus, and hamstrings). Hold a relatively light weight and slowly flex the shoulders through full range of motion (upper arm near ear), control descent of the weight to the starting position.

Bent-over lateral raise (DB): Feet shoulder width apart, knees slightly flexed, hips flexed to 90 degrees, chest and chin up, and keep torso stable (contract abdominals, gluteus, and hamstrings). Hold a relatively light weight and horizontally abduct the shoulders slowly through full range of motion (squeeze shoulder blades together). Control descent of the weight to starting position.

Bent-over row (barbell): Feet shoulder width apart, knees slightly flexed, hips flexed to 90 degrees. Arms are extended and hold the barbell toward the floor. Exhale while flexing the elbows and pulling the bar to the chest. Control descent of the weight to starting position.

Box jumps: See plyometric descriptions and figures.

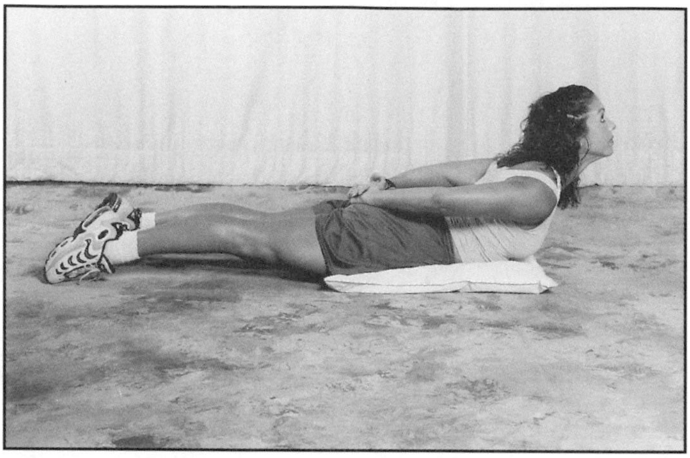

Figure A-1. Back extension on floor.

Close grip bench press (barbell): Straddle the bench, feet on the ground, knees flexed to 90 degrees. Head, shoulders, and hips on the bench at all times; overhand grip should be just inside shoulder width. Keep wrists tight and in line with the elbows, inhale and, with control, lower the barbell/DB to the breast line. Exhale while pushing upward and back to eye level. Barbell/DB should execute a slightly curved descent and ascent, keep the elbows close to the body through range of motion. At completion of ascent, wrists should still be in line with extended elbows.

Close grip push-up (body weight): Hands on the floor slightly inside shoulder width, head and neck in neutral position, torso stable, knees extended, and feet on the floor shoulder width apart. Inhale while descending the body slowly to the ground; keep elbows close to the body and exhale during ascent.

Curl, biceps (E-Z bar/DB/barbell/cable, standing/seated/incline): Feet shoulder width apart, knees slightly flexed, torso stable, eyes forward, upper arms and elbows secure to the side, slightly supinate the forearms and slowly flex and extend the elbows through full range of motion.

Dead lift (barbell): Barbell close to shins, feet just inside shoulder width, knees flexed, overhand or alternating grip just outside the knees, stable torso, shoulders over the knees and higher than the hips, eyes and chin up and forward. Exhale as the hips and knees extend simultaneously, keep the barbell close to the body, elbows extended and torso stable. Inhale as the barbell is lowered to the floor slowly (Figures A-2a, A-2b).

Decline push-up (body weight): Hands on the floor wider than shoulder width, head and neck in neutral position, torso stable, knees extended, feet elevated 12 inches to 24 inches. Inhale while descending the body (chin) slowly to the ground, exhale during ascent.

Dips (body weight): Hands on the apparatus shoulder width apart, elbows extended, keep the torso stable, inhale as the elbows are slowly flexed to 90 degrees and kept close to the body; allow chest to fall forward slightly, and exhale as elbows are extended fully.

Flys (DB, lying/incline): Straddle the bench, feet on the ground, knees flexed to 90 degrees, head, shoulders, and hips on the bench at all times. Gripping the weight with slightly pronated forearms (palms facing each other), horizontally abduct and adduct the weight, finishing together at chest level for lying and eye level for incline.

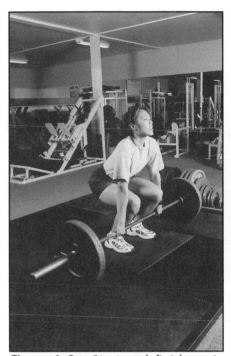

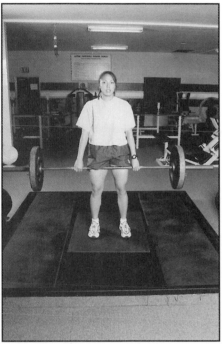

Figure A-2a. Start and finish position of dead lift.

Figure A-2b. Extension position of dead lift.

Front raise (DB/barbell/cable): Feet shoulder width apart, knees slightly flexed, torso stable, eyes forward, grip the weight with an overhand grip, flex (raise/lift) the shoulders to 90 degrees and control descent.

Front squat (barbell): Feet slightly wider than shoulder width, barbell positioned on the anterior deltoids in a clean-catch arm position. Eyes and chin are up and forward. Inhale, unlock and slowly flex the hips to 90 degrees, keep the torso stable, chest and eyes up, body weight on the heels, knees over the toes, and elbows up. During the ascent, exhale while driving the hips up and extending the knees fully (Figure A-3).

Good mornings (barbell): Feet slightly wider than shoulder width, keep the knees slightly flexed, torso stable, eyes forward, and barbell positioned on the posterior deltoids. Hold this position and inhale while flexing the hips to 90 degrees. Exhale and extend to an upright position.

Hammer curl (DB, standing/seated/incline): Feet shoulder width apart, knees slightly flexed, torso stable, eyes forward, gripping the weight with 90-degree pronated forearms (hammer position), secure the upper arms and elbows to the side, slowly flex and extend the elbows fully.

Hang clean (DB/barbell): Feet shoulder width apart, overhand grip just outside the knees, torso stable, and standing erect (holding weight). Exhale as the barbell/DB lowers to the knees with the shoulders over the flexed knees and higher than the hips, eyes forward. Inhale and pull the barbell/DB quickly and closely to the body as the hips drive up and forward, knees extend fully, ankles plantarflex (as in a vertical jump), shoulders shrug and pull (flex elbows

Figure A-3. Descent position of front squat.

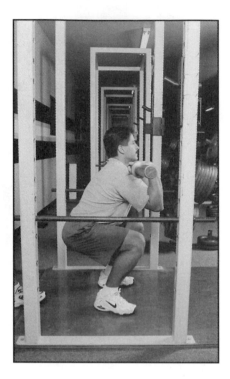

out wide with the barbell after maximal shrug), close to the body. As barbell/DB reaches shoulder height (body drops under bar), hips and knees flex, ankles dorsiflex, body weight is on the heels, elbows are rotated under the barbell/DB (parallel to the floor) and barbell/DB is caught on the anterior deltoids. Holding the catch position, hips and knees extend to an upright position. The barbell/DB is lowered to the knees in a controlled manner (Figures A-4a, A-4b).

Hang snatch (barbell): Feet shoulder width apart, hold with an overhand grip wide at the knees, stable torso, shoulders over the flexed knees and higher than the hips, eyes forward. Exhale as the bar is pulled close to the body, elbows are extended at this point, hips and knees extend simultaneously. As the barbell passes the hips, hold your breath slightly and pull the bar quickly and closely to the body as the hips drive up and forward, knees extend fully, ankles plantarflex (as in a vertical jump), and shoulders shrug (flex elbows out wide after maximal shrug). As the barbell reaches shoulder height (body drops under barbell), hips and knees flex, ankles dorsiflex, weight is on the heels, shoulders externally rotate, and the barbell is caught overhead with elbows extended. Holding the catch position, the hips and knees extend to an upright position. The barbell is lowered to the knees and then to the floor in a controlled manner (Figures A-5a, A5b).

High pull (barbell): Feet shoulder width apart, overhand grip just outside the knees, torso stable, and standing erect (holding the weight). Exhale as the bar lowers to the knees with the shoulders over the flexed knees and higher than hips, eyes forward. Inhale and pull bar quickly and closely to the body as the hips drive up and forward, knees extend fully, ankles plantarflex, shoulders shrug, and pull (flex elbows out wide after maximal shrug) barbell close to body. As the barbell reaches eye level, the body drops as the bar is suspended and, simultaneously, the hips and knees flex, ankles dorsiflex, and weight is on the heels. There is no catch

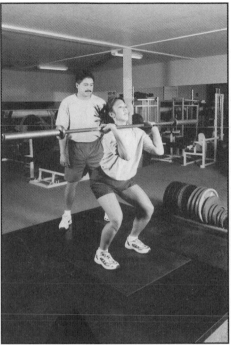

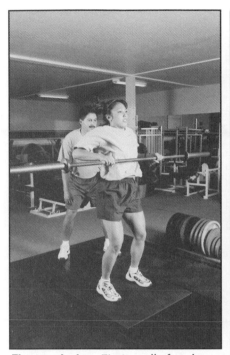

Figure A-4a. First pull for hang clean, second pull for power clean.

Figure A-4b. Catch position for hang and power clean

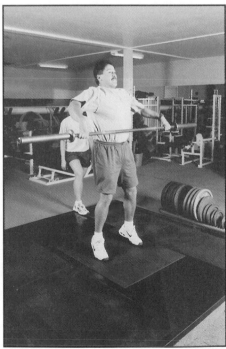

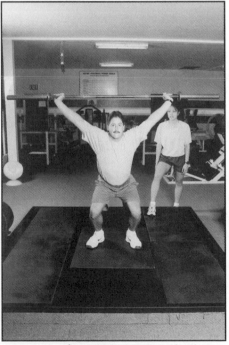

Figure A-5a. First pull for hang snatch, second pull for power snatch.

Figure A-5b. Catch position for hang and power snatch.

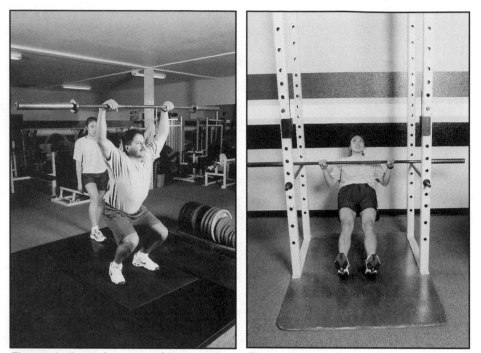

Figure A-6. High point of high pull.   **Figure A-7.** Incline pull-up position.

at the top, and the weight is brought back to the knees in a controlled manner (Figure A-6).

Hip routine: See descriptions and figures.

Ice skaters: See plyometric descriptions and figures.

Incline press (DB/barbell): Straddle the bench, feet on the ground, knees flexed to 90 degrees, head, shoulders, and hips on the bench at all times, overhand grip wider than shoulder width. Keep wrists tight and in line with the elbows. Inhale and, with control, lower the barbell/DB to the upper chest (clavicle), exhale while pushing upward and back to eye level. Barbell/DB should execute a slightly curved descent and ascent. At completion of ascent, the wrists should still be in line with the extended elbows.

Incline push-up (body weight): Hands elevated 12 inches to 24 inches (prone position) wider than shoulder width, head and neck in neutral position, torso stable, knees extended, feet shoulder width apart on the floor. Inhale while descending the body (chest) slowly to the bar/bench, exhale during ascent.

Incline pull up (body weight): Apparatus is elevated 24 inches to 36 inches (supine position), hands grasp the bar wider than shoulder width, head and neck in neutral, torso stable, knees extended, feet/heels shoulder width on the floor, inhale while pulling the body (chest) to the barbell, exhale during controlled descent. Do not allow the hips to sag during exercise (Figure A-7).

Jump rope routine: See plyometric description.

Ladder: See description.

Lat pull-down (overhand/underhand, close/wide, universal): Using a variety of grips, straddle the bench, feet on the floor, slowly pull the bar to the upper chest, keep the torso stable, control the bar to starting position.

Lateral box/cone jumps: See plyometric descriptions and figures.

Lateral raise (DB/cable): Feet shoulder width apart, knees slightly flexed, torso stable, eyes forward, grip the weight with the palms facing each other, abduct (raise/lift) the shoulders to 90 degrees and control descent.

Leg extension (single/double, universal): Seated, torso stable, eyes forward, and extend the knees fully. Externally rotate the hip to emphasize vastus medialis and internally rotate the hip to emphasize vastus lateralis.

Leg curl (single/double, universal): Prone, hips stable, and flex knees fully. Externally rotate the leg to emphasize the biceps femoris, internally rotate the leg to emphasize semitendinosus and semimembranosus.

Leg sled (machine): Supine; neck, shoulders, and hips on the bench. Hips flexed to 45 degrees, feet secure on the pedals, inhale and flex the hips and knees (90 degrees). Exhale and push the knees to full extension. Place the feet high on the pedals to emphasize the hamstrings.

Lunge (DB/barbell): Toes pointed forward, torso and hips stable, eyes forward; step forward, flex the hip and knee (90 degrees) to position (knee) over the toes, the stationary knee should flex in order to center the weight. Push back with the forward foot to the halfway position, then step together. This will decrease use of momentum. Step forward with the opposite leg (Figure A-8).

Lunge, lateral (body weight/barbell): Toes pointed forward, torso stable, eyes forward, abduct the leg (step wide to side), keep the stationary knee extended, flex the lunging knee and keep it over the toes that are pointing forward. Adduct (pull) the leg to its original position and perform with the opposite leg (Figure A-9).

Lunge, 4-way (body weight/barbell): Lunge forward (see lunge), lunge to the side (see lateral lunge), lunge at a 45 degree angle (between forward and lateral lunge position), lunge as the right leg crosses (toes forward, knee over the toes, and body weight is at the center) over the stationary leg (left) at a 45 degree angle for one set.

Lunge squat (DB/barbell): Hold a lunge descent position and extend both knees, squat (descend) and extend (ascend) in this position.

Lying tricep extension (DB): Straddle the bench in supine position, feet on the ground, knees flexed to 90 degrees, head, shoulders, and hips on the bench at all times, gripping the weight (hammer position), flex the shoulders to approximately 140 degrees and hold. From this position, slowly extend and flex the elbows fully.

Medicine ball abdominal: See abdominal descriptions and figures.

Medicine ball exercises: See medicine ball descriptions and figures.

Military press (DB/barbell, standing/seated): Feet shoulder width apart, knees slightly flexed, torso stable, eyes forward, and grip the weight with an overhand grip. Flex the elbows and bring the weight to shoulder height (palms facing forward). Exhale as the shoulders simultaneously abduct with elbow extension. The weight should finish overhead; inhale during controlled descent of the weight.

Neck, 4-way (machine): Seated on apparatus, feet on floor, keep torso stable as neck (only) flexes, extends, and laterally flexes in both directions.

One-arm row (DB): Unilateral hand and knee on the bench, opposite leg extended with the foot on the floor. Begin holding the weight perpendicular to the floor, hyperextend the

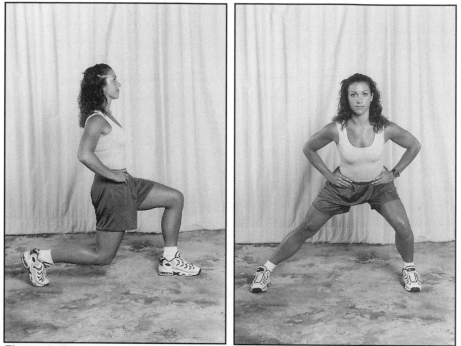

Figure A-8. Lunge position.   **Figure A-9.** Lateral lunge position.

shoulder as the elbow flexes (close to body), pulling the weight to the side of the torso. Control the weight to the starting position.

Power clean (barbell): Barbell on the floor close to the shins, feet shoulder width apart, overhand grip just outside the knees, stable torso, the shoulders over flexed knees and higher than the hips, eyes forward. Exhale as the bar is pulled close to the body, elbows are extended at this point, hips and knees extend simultaneously. As the barbell passes the knees, hold your breath slightly and the pull bar quickly and closely to the body as the hips drive up and forward, the knees extend fully, ankles plantarflex (as in a vertical jump), and the shoulders shrug (flex the elbows out wide after a maximal shrug). As the barbell reaches shoulder height (body drops under barbell), the hips and knees flex, ankles dorsiflex, weight is on the heels, elbows are rotated under the barbell (parallel to the floor) and the barbell is caught on the anterior deltoids. Holding the catch position, the hips and knees extend to an upright position. The barbell is lowered to the knees and then to the floor in a controlled manner (refer to hang clean in Figures A-4a, A-4b).

Power shrug (barbell): Feet shoulder width apart, knees slightly flexed, torso stable, eyes forward, and grip the weight with an overhand grip. The barbell lowers over the thighs as the hips flex slightly. The shoulders then forcefully shrug as the hips and knees extend. The elbow stay extended through the exercise.

Power snatch (barbell): Barbell on the floor close to the shins, feet shoulder width apart, overhand grip wide outside the knees, stable torso, shoulders over the flexed knees and higher than the hips, eyes forward. Exhale as the bar is pulled close to the body, elbows are extended at this point, hips and knees extend simultaneously. As the barbell passes the knees, hold

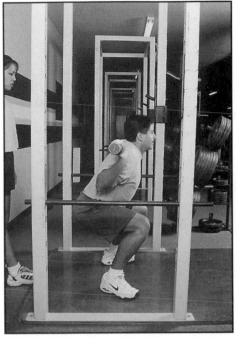

Figure A-10. Descent position of power squat.

your breath slightly and pull the bar quickly and closely to the body as the hips drive up and forward, knees extend fully, ankles plantarflex (as in a vertical jump), and shoulders shrug (flex the elbows out wide after maximal shrug). As the barbell reaches shoulder height (body drops under barbell), hips and knees flex, ankles dorsiflex, weight is on the heels, shoulders externally rotate, and barbell is caught overhead with the elbows extended. Holding the catch position, the hips and knees extend to an upright position. The barbell is lowered to the knees and then to the floor in a controlled manner (refer to hang snatch in Figures A-5a, A-5b)

Power squat (barbell): Feet shoulder width apart, torso stable, barbell held on the posterior deltoids, and eyes forward. Inhale and hold the breath slightly. Flex the hips and knees (90 degrees), keeping the chest and eyes up. Exhale during ascent as the hips and knees extend fully (Figure A-10).

Prone neck extension (body weight): Prone on the bench (head is off) with the hands behind the back for beginners; working toward the back of the head for advanced. Slowly extend and flex the head/neck.

Pullover (E-Z bar/DB/barbell/cable): Straddle the bench in supine position, feet on the ground, knees flexed to 90 degrees, head, shoulders, and hips on the bench at all times. With an overhand grip and slightly flexed elbows, flex and extend the shoulders fully allowing weight to pass behind the head.

Pull-up (overhand/underhand, close/wide, body weight): Gripping the apparatus using a variety of grips, keep the torso stable and pull/lift the body as the chin passes. Attempt to keep the legs from moving.

Push press (DB/barbell): Standing with feet shoulder width apart (staggered or side by side), knees slightly flexed, torso stable, eyes forward, and grip the weight with an overhand grip. Flex the elbows and bring the weight to shoulder height (palms facing forward). Exhale

Figure A-11. Catch position of push press.

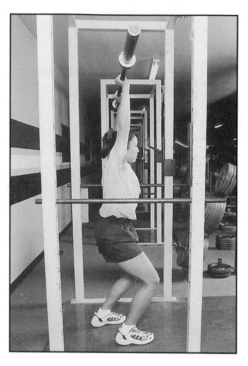

as the hips and knees flex and the shoulders simultaneously abduct with elbow extension. Weight should finish overhead elbows; hips and knees are extended. Inhale during controlled descent of weight (Figure A-11).

Rear deltoid pull (universal): Standing with the feet shoulder width apart and staggered for support, grip the weight from a position above the eyes and pull to the face as the shoulders horizontally abduct and elbows flex. Squeeze the scapulae together and control the weight to its starting position.

Rear military press (barbell, seated): Straddle the bench, feet shoulder width apart on the floor, knees flexed, torso stable, eyes forward, and grip the weight with an overhand grip. Flex the elbows and bring the weight behind the neck on the posterior deltoids (palms facing forward). Exhale as the shoulders simultaneously abduct with elbow extension. The weight should finish overhead; inhale during controlled descent of the weight.

Reverse back extension (body weight): On a back extension apparatus, grip the ankle supports with the hands and place the hips on the pad. Extend the hips to parallel while maintaining a stable torso. Control descent of the legs to their starting position.

Reverse lateral raise (DB): Standing with the feet shoulder width apart, knees slightly flexed, torso stable, eyes forward, grip the weight with the palms facing each other, abduct (raise/lift) the shoulders to 90 degrees, externally rotate the shoulders and continue abduction to 180 degrees. The weight should be overhead and the palms facing each other. Internally rotate at 90 degrees during descent and finish with the palms facing each other.

Reverse lunge (barbell): Toes pointed forward, torso and hips stable, eyes forward, step backward, extend the moving hip to allow the stationary hip to flex (90 degrees) and the knee (90 degrees) to position over the toes. Push forward with the back foot to step together. Step back with the opposite leg.

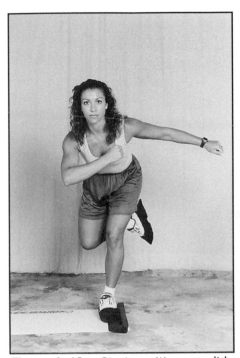 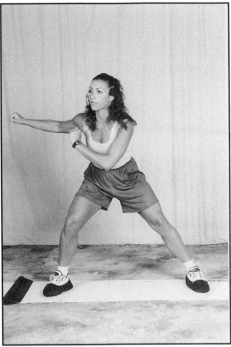

Figure A-12a. Start position on slide board. **Figure A-12b.** Slide form on slide board.

Rice routine: See supplemental routine description.

Rotator cuff warm-up routine: See description.

Seated calves (machine): Seated, torso stable, middle of feet on apparatus, and the knees flexed to 90 degrees, plantarflex the ankles. Toes may be positioned in, straight, or out.

Seated row (universal): Seated, torso stable, shoulders flexed, elbows extended, and knees slightly flexed. Extend the back to an upright position while pulling the weight to the mid torso. Keep the elbows in and squeeze the scapulae together.

Shrug (DB): Feet shoulder width apart, dumbbells held at each side with extended elbows. Shrug shoulders fully while maintaining extended elbows.

Single-leg 6-Inch box jumps: See plyometric description.

Single-leg speed hops: See plyometric description.

Slide board: Eyes forward, weight mostly on the starting leg, torso stable, hips, knees, and elbows slightly flexed. Push against the stationary stopper on the board while pushing out with the other. The opposite arm should move with the leg in a speed skater type motion. The body should propel across the board in one smooth movement. Repeat on the other side, allowing only enough time for following leg to get in position to push again (Figures A-12a, A-12b).

Squat (DB): Feet shoulder width apart, torso stable, dumbbells held at each side with extended elbows, and eyes forward. Inhale and hold your breath slightly. Flex the hips and knees (90 degrees), keeping the chest and eyes up. Exhale during ascent as the hips and knees extend fully.

Squat jump (body weight/DB): Feet shoulder width apart, torso stable, dumbbells held at

Figure A-13a. Squat (start and finish) position of squat jump.

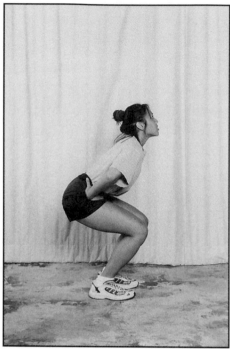

each side with extended elbows and eyes forward. Inhale and hold your breath slightly. Flex the hips and knees (90 degrees), keeping the chest and eyes up, jump straight up in the air. Land with flexed knees to absorb impact (Figures A-13a, A-13b).

Standing calves (single/double, body weight/DB/machine): Standing with support, plantarflex the ankles fully. The toes may be positioned in, straight, or out.

Step up (UE), lower extremity (forward/lateral, body weight/DB/barbell): Using an elevated surface (12 inches to 18 inches), step up so that the entire foot is on the surface. The thigh should be parallel to the floor, torso stable, and eyes forward. Extend the hip and knee to bring the stationary leg up to the elevated surface. Now step down with either the same leg or the opposite leg. (Figure A-14).

Step up, upper extremity (body weight): Using an elevated surface (6 inches to 10 inches), step up so that the entire hand is on the surface. The torso, hips, and legs should be stable in a push-up position. Step up with the stationary hand so both hands are on the elevated surface. Step down with the same hand or the opposite hand. (Figures A-15a, A-15b).

Stiff-leg dead lift (DB/barbell): Torso stable, knees very slightly flexed, head and eyes remain looking forward. Lower the weight slowly and close to the body until it touches the floor. Be very careful not to round the back and allow the head and neck to flex forward. Concentrate on contracting the glutes and hamstrings to avoid low-back injury, while extending the back to an upright position.

Straight Lat pull-down (overhand/underhand, universal): Standing, facing lat pull-down apparatus, feet wider than shoulder width, torso stable, and grip bar with extended elbows. Keep the elbows extended through the exercise and pull the bar down toward the thighs. Control the weight to its starting position.

Supine neck flexion (body weight/weight plate): Straddle the bench, feet on the ground,

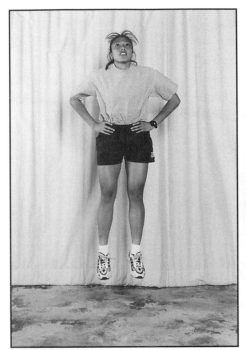

Figure A-13b. Jump position of squat jump.

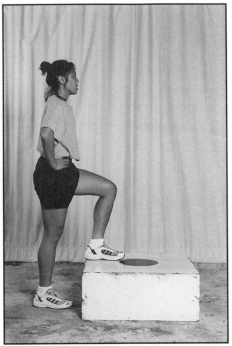

Figure A-14. Lower extremity step up position.

knees flexed to 90 degrees, shoulders and hips on the bench at all times, and arms crossed across the chest or holding a weight plate. Slowly flex and extend the neck.

T-bar row (overhand/underhand, machine): Feet shoulder width apart on the T-bar apparatus, knees slightly flexed, hips flex so the torso is just above parallel with the floor. Arms are extended and hold the bar toward floor. Exhale while flexing the elbows and pulling the bar to the chest. Control descent of weight to starting position. Be careful not to allow the low back to round, keep glutes and hamstrings contracted through the exercise.

Torso twist: See abdominal program.

Towel pull-up: Gripping the apparatus using a towel, pull/lift the body and pull the towel in toward your shoulders. The hands (grip) should be in hammer position and kept very close to the body.

Tricep extension (DB): Standing, torso stable, eyes forward, feet shoulder width apart, and knees slightly flexed. Raise the weight behind the head so the shoulders are flexed to approximately 170 degrees and elbows are flexed. Hold this position and extend and flex the elbows. Weight should stay behind the head through the exercise.

Tricep kickback (DB): Unilateral hand and knee on the bench, opposite leg extended with the foot on the floor. Moving arm, hyperextended, remains with the shoulder. From this position, extend and flex the elbow in a controlled manner.

Tricep push-down (overhand/underhand, single/double, universal): Standing, torso stable, feet shoulder width apart, knees slightly flexed, and eyes forward. Keep the upper arms and elbows secure next to the torso through the exercise. Extend and flex the elbows slowly.

Twisting back extension (body weight): Prone on the floor (pad/pillow under the hips) or

Figure A-15a. Start position of upper extremity step up.

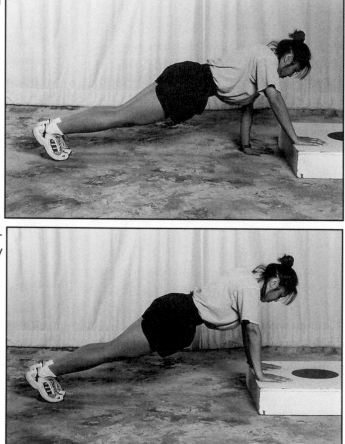

Figure A-15b. Mid-point position of upper extremity stepup.

apparatus, hands behind the back for beginners, work hands toward head for advanced, torso stable and feet secure. Extend the back as it rotates to one side and until the chest is no longer touching the floor or parallel with the floor if on the apparatus, control descent. Repeat, extend, and rotate the other side for one repetition.

Upright row (DB/barbell/cable): Standing, torso stable, feet shoulder width apart, knees slightly flexed, and eyes forward. Overhand grip the weight close so the hands are approximately three inches apart. Keeping the weight close to the body (so the elbows will flex wide), pull the weight up to the chin and return to the starting position slowly.

Walking lunges (body weight/DB): Toes pointed forward, torso and hips stable, eyes forward, step forward, flex the hip and knee (90 degrees) to position (knee) over the toes, the stationary knee should flex in order to center the weight. Extend, then moving (now stationary), the hip and knee to bring the stationary (now moving) leg forward. Keep the chest up and do not bend forward to accomplish this. Shorten the step if this happens. Step out with the opposite leg moving forward.

Wrist extension (DB/barbell): Stabilize the pronated forearm on the bench. Allow the wrist to extend and flex fully.

Wrist flexion (DB/barbell): Stabilize the supinated forearm on the bench. Allow the wrist to flex and extend fully.

Bibliography

Adler S, Beckrs D, Buck M. *PNF and Practice: An Illustrated Guide.* 2nd ed. New York: Springer Publisher; 2000.

American Academy of Pediatrics. Policy statement: Human immunodeficiency virus (acquired immunodeficiency syndrome [AIDS] virus) in the athletic setting. *Pediatrics.* 1991;88:640-641.

American Academy of Pediatrics (Committee on Sports Medicine). Policy statement: Amenorrhea in adolescent athletes. *Pediatrics.* 1989;84:394-395.

American Academy of Pediatrics (Committee on Sports Medicine). Policy statement: Strength training, weight and power lifting, and body building by children and adolescents. *Pediatrics.* 1990;86:801-803.

American College of Sports Medicine (ACSM). *ACSM's Exercise Management for Persons with Chronic Diseases and Disabilities.* Champaign, Ill: Human Kinetics; 1997.

American College of Sports Medicine (ACSM). *ACSM's Guidelines for Exercise Testing and Prescriptions.* 5th ed. Philadelphia, Pa: Williams & Wilkins; 1995.

American College of Sports Medicine (ACSM). Position stand on exercise and fluid replacement. *Med Sci Sports Exerc.* 1996;28:i-vii.

American Council on Exercise. *Clinical Exercise Specialist Manual: ACE's Source for Training Special Populations.* ACE, 1999.

American Diabetes Association. *The Health Professional's Guide to Diabetes and Exercise.* ADA; 1995.

Armstrong LE, Costill DL, Fink WJ. Influence of diuretic-induced dehydration on competitive running performance. *Med Sci Sports Exerc.* 1985;17:456-461.

Anderson B. *Stretching.* Bolinas, CA: Shelter Publications, Inc; 1980.

Askew EW. *Nutrition in Exercise and Sport.* 3rd ed. Boca Raton, Fl: CRC Press LLC; 1998.

Baechle TR, Groves BR. *Weight Training, Steps to Success.* Champaign, Ill: Leisure Press; 1992.

Below P, Mora-Rodriguez R, Gonzalez-Alonso J, Coyle EF. Fluid and carbohydrate ingestion independently improve performance during 1 h of intense exercise. *Med Sci Sports Exerc.* 1995;27:200-210.

Borkowski, RP. Safety for the weight room. *Fitness Management Magazine.* 1999;15:44.

Brooks GA, Fahey TD, White TP. *Exercise Physiology: Human Bioenergetics and its Applications.* 2nd ed. Mountain View, Calif: Mayfield Publishing Company; 1996.

Bryant DX, Peterson JA. Not for adults only. *Fitness Management Magazine.* 1996;12:34-36.

Bucci LR. *Nutrition in Exercise and Sport.* 3rd ed. Boca Raton, Fl: CRC Press LLC; 1998.

Burr DB. Bone, exercise, and stress fractures. *Exercise and Sport Science Reviews.* 1997;25:171-194.

Butterfield G. Ergogenic aids: evaluating sport nutrition products. *Int J of Sport Nutr.* 1996;6:191-197.

CDC. Center for Disease Control and Prevention web site. Available at www.cdc.gov. Accessed 1997.

Chu, DA. *Jumping into Plyometrics.* 2nd ed. Champaign, Ill: Human Kinetics; 1998.

Chu D, Plummer L. The language of plyometrics. *National Strength and Conditioning Association Journal.* 1984;6:63-64.

Corbin CB, Pangrazi RP. *Toward a Better Understanding of Physical Fitness & Activity.* Scottsdale, Ariz: Holcomb Hathaway Publishers; 1999.

Dick FW. *Sports Training Principles.* 3rd ed. London: A&C Black Publishers; 1997.

DiFiori JP. Overuse injuries in children and adolescents. *The Physician and Sportsmedicine.* 1999;27.

Duda M. Prepubescent strength training gains support. *The Physician and Sportsmedicine.* 1986;14:157-161.

Grabiner MD, Enoka RM. Changes in movement capabilities with aging. *Exercise and Sport Science Reviews.* 1995;23:65-104.

Groziak SM, Miller GD. *Nutrition in Exercise and Sport.* 3rd ed. Boca Raton, Fl: CRC Press LLC; 1998.

Grunewald KK, Bailey RS. Commercially marketed supplements for bodybuilding athletes. *Sports Med.* 1993;15:90-103.

Herbert DL. Failure to spot may constitute misconduct. *Fitness Management Magazine.* 1996;12:21.

Herbert DL. Costly failure to provide emergency response. *Fitness Management Magazine.* 1996;12:24.

Herbert DL. Managing risk. *Fitness Management Magazine.* 1997;13:45-47.

Herbert DL. Spotter may be liable for injury. *Fitness Management Magazine.* 1998;14:52.

Herbert DL. Waiver upheld for California facility. *Fitness Management Magazine.* 1999;15:46.

Horswill CA. Effective fluid replacement. *Int J Sport Nutr.* 1998;8:175-195.

Jeukendrup A, Brouns F, Wagenmakers AJ, Saris WH. Carbohydrate-electrolyte feedings improve 1 h time trial cycling performance. *Int J Sports Med.* 1997;18:125-129.

Kibler WB, Chandler TJ, Stracener ES. Musculoskeletal adaptations and injuries due to overtraining. *Exercise and Sport Science Reviews.* 1992;20:99-126.

Kisner C & Colby LA. *Therapeutic Exercise: Foundations and Techniques.* Philadelphia, Pa:. FA Davis; 1990.

Kris-Etherton PM. The facts and fallacies of nutritional supplements for athletes. *Gatorade Sports Science Exchange.* 1989;2:18.

Lemon P. Do athletes need more dietary protein and amino acids? *Int J Sport Nutr.* 1995;5:S39-S61.

Marquart LF, Cohen EA, Short SH. *Nutrition in Exercise and Sport.* 3rd ed. Boca Raton, Fl: CRC Press LLC; 1998.

Micheli LJ, Jenkins M. The sports medicine bible. *Strength and Flexibility: The Key to Injury Prevention.* New York, NY: Harper Collins Publishers; 1995.

McFarlane B. A look inside the biomechanics and dynamics of speed. *National Strength and Conditioning Association Journal.* 1987;9:35-45.

National Strength & Conditioning Association. *Essentials of Strength Training and Conditioning.* Champaign, Ill: Human Kinetics; 1994.

Nelson WE. *Behrman: Nelson Texbook of Pediatrics.* 15th ed. Philadelphia, Pa: WB Saunders Company; 1996.

Nicholas CW, Williams C, Phillips G, Nowitz A. Influence of ingesting a carbohydrate-electrolyte solution on endurance capacity during intermittent, high intensity shuttle running. *J Sports Sci.* 1996;13:283-290.

Passe D, Horn M, Murray R. The effects of beverage carbonation on sensory responses and voluntary fluid intake following exercise. *Int J Sport Nutr.* 1997;7:286-297.

Paul G. Dietary protein requirements of physically active individuals. *Sports Med.* 1989;8:154-176.

Perrin DH. *Isokinetic Exercise & Assessment.* Champaign, Ill: Human Kinetics; 1993.

Picone RE. Strength training for children. *Fitness Management Magazine.* 1999;15:32-35.

Pizza FX, Flynn MG, Duscha BD, Holman J, Kubitz ER. A carbohydrate-loading regimen improves high intensity, short duration exercise performance. *Int J Sport Nutr.* 1995;5:110-116.

Pollock ML, Wilmore JH. *Exercise in Health and Disease.* 2nd ed. Philadelphia, Pa: WB Saunders Company; 1990.

Powers SK, Howley ET. *Exercise Physiology.* 3rd ed. Dubuque, Iowa: Brown & Benchmark Publishers; 1997.

Rock CL. *Nutrition in Exercise and Sport.* 3rd ed. Boca Raton, Fl: CRC Press LLC; 1998.

Rogers MA, Evans WJ. Changes in skeletal muscle with aging: Effects of exercise training. *American College of Sports Medicine Series: Exercise and Sport Science Reviews.* 1993;21:65-102.

Roy S, Irvin R. *Sports Medicine: Prevention, Evaluation, Management & Rehabilitation.* Englewood Cliffs, NJ: Prentice-Hall, Inc; 1983.

Ruud JS, Grandjean AC. *Nutrition in Exercise and Sport.* 3rd ed. Boca Raton, Fl: CRC Press LLC; 1998.

Schafer J. Prepubescent and adolescent weight training: Is it safe? Is it beneficial? *National Strength and Conditioning Association Journal.* 1991;13:39-46.

Schnirring L. With Magic back, what are the medical messages? *The Physician and Sportsmedicine.* 1996;24:27-28.

Sherman WM, Costill DL, Fink WJ, Miller JM. The effect of exercise and diet manipulation on muscle glycogen and its subsequent utilization during performance. *Int J Sports Med.* 1981;2:114-118.

Staver P. Dispelling the myths of children & weights. *Fitness Management Magazine.* 1996;12:43-44.

Stephenson LA, Kolka MA. Thermoregulation in women. *Exercise and Sport Science Reviews.* 1993;21:231-262.

Stone WJ, Kroll WA. *Sports conditioning and weight training, programs for athletic competition.* 3rd ed. Dubuque, IA; 1988.

Sundgot-Borgen J. Prevalence of eating disorders in elite female athletes. *Int J Sport Nutr.* 1993;3:29-41.

Sundgot-Borgen J. Risk and trigger factors for the development of eating disorders in female elite athletes. *Med Sci Sports Exerc.* 1994;26:414-419.

Tarnopolsky M. Protein, caffeine, and sports. Guidelines for active people. *Phys and Sportsmed.* 1993;21:137-149.

US Department of Agriculture, Human Nutrition Information Service. *Nutrition and Your Health: Dietary Guidelines for Americans.* 4th ed. Washington, DC: US Government Printing Office; 1995.

US Department of Agriculture, Human Nutrition Information Service. *The Food Guide Pyramid. Home and Garden Bulletin Number 252.* Washington, DC: US Government Printing Office; 1995.

Vega, J. Shifting the exercise mode to sporty. *Fitness Management Magazine.* 1997;13:45-47.

Wallberg-Henriksson H. Exercise and diabetes mellitus. *American College of Sports Medicine Series: Exercise and Sport Science Reviews.* 1992;20:339-368.

Walsh RM, Noakes TD, Hawley JA, Dennis SC. Impaired high-intensity cycling performance time at low levels of dehydration. *Int J Sports Med.* 1994;15:392-398.

Ward PE, Ward RD. *Encyclopedia of Weight Training: Weight Training for General Conditioning, Sport and Body Building.* Laguna Hills, CA: QPT Publications; 1991.

Whitehill WR, Wright KE. AIDS: Guidelines for the athletic community. *National Strength and Conditioning Association Journal.* 1990;12:64-67.

Williams MH. *Nutrition for Health, Fitness, & Sport.* 5th ed. Dubuque, Iowa: WCB McGraw-Hill; 1999.

Williams MH. Nutritional supplements for strength trained athletes. *Gatorade Sports Science Exchange.* 1993;6:47.

Williams MH. The use of nutritional ergogenic aids in sports: is it an ethical issue? *Int J Sport Nutr.* 1994;4:120-131.

Wilmore JH. *Professional Preparation in Athletic Training.* Champaign, Ill: Human Kinetics, 1982.

Zatsiorsky VM. *Science and Practice of Strength Training.* Champaign, Il: Human Kinetics; 1995.

Index

machine whole body circuits, 150–151
macrocycle, 27
maximum heart rate, 65, 70
maximum oxygen consumption, 65
medical history, 69
Medicine and Science in Sports and Exercise, 102
medicine ball routines, 146–148, 150, 151
menstrual cycle, 83
mesocycle, 27–28
metabolic equivalent levels (METs), 71
microcycles, 29
motivation, 36
multijoint exercises, 30, 37
multijoint lifts, 27
muscle action velocity, 22
muscle cross-sectional area, 21
muscle fibers, arrangement of, 21
muscle force, 21
muscle imbalance, overuse, 125
muscle length, 21–22
muscle mass, 49
muscle performance
    isokinetic, 20–21
    isometric, 19
    isotonic, 20
    principles of, 19–22
muscle spindle, 112–113
musculoskeletal system, 21
myocardium, 57
myotatic reflex, 41

neck stabilization routine, 133–135
National Athletic Trainers' Association (NATA), 6–8
National Council for Reliable Health Information (NCRHI), 103
National Strength and Conditioning Association (NSCA), 3–4, 14, 28
negligence, legal claims of, 13
neural control, 21
nutrition, 59–60. *See also diet*

olympic lifting, 38, 121–122, 124–125

one-mile walk test, 69
over distance training, 65
overtraining, 125
overuse injury, 125–126
oxygen
    partial pressure of, 58–59
    tissue exchange of, 58–59
    transport and exchange of, 57
oxyhemoglobin, 58–59

Parks vs. Gilligan, 14
participants, safety and legal issues of, 15
pediatric sports injuries, 45–46
periodization, 27–31
phosphates, 60
physical examination program, pre-participation, 69
physical maturity, assessment of, 47
physician clearance, 69
pivot point, 21
plantar facitis, 117
plyometric drills, 30
plyometric training, 42–43, 76
    warm-up period for, 42
plyometrics, 29, 41
    lower extremity, 140–146
    phases of, 41–42
    prescription for, 42–43
    principles of, 41
potential energy, 41
power, 21
power lifting, 123–124
pre-exhaustion sets, 29
pregame meals, 95
prepubescent athletes, 45–48
professional organizations, 3–10
progressive resistive exercises, 26–27
    daily adjustable, 27
proprioceptive neuromuscular facilitation (PNF), 111, 112–114
protein, 59–60
    metabolism of in seniors, 49
    recommended intake of, 93
pulmonary capacity, 58